365 Days of Ketogenic Diet Recipes

Over 50 Tasty Diet Recipes to Make Every Day

© **Copyright 2021 All rights reserved.**

This document is geared towards providing exact and reliable information with regards to the topic and issue covered. The publication is sold with the idea that the publisher is not required to render accounting, officially permitted, or otherwise, qualified services. If advice is necessary, legal or professional, a practiced individual in the profession should be ordered.

From a Declaration of Principles which was accepted and approved equally by a Committee of the American Bar Association and a Committee of Publishers and Associations.

In no way is it legal to reproduce, duplicate, or transmit any part of this document in either electronic means or in printed format. Recording of this publication is strictly prohibited and any storage of this document is not allowed unless with written permission from the publisher. All rights reserved.

The information provided herein is stated to be truthful and consistent, in that any liability, in terms of inattention or otherwise, by any usage or abuse of any policies, processes, or directions contained within is the solitary and utter responsibility of the recipient reader. Under no circumstances will any legal responsibility or blame be held against the publisher for any reparation, damages, or monetary loss due to the information herein, either directly or indirectly.

Respective authors own all copyrights not held by the publisher.

The information herein is offered for informational purposes solely, and is universal as so. The presentation of the information is without contract or any type of guarantee assurance.

The trademarks that are used are without any consent, and the publication of the trademark is without permission or backing by the trademark owner. All trademarks and brands within this book are for clarifying purposes only and are the owned by the owners themselves, not affiliated with this document

CONTENTS

Introduction 7
THE KETOSIS 10
DIET – THE NEW LIFESTYLE 15
BASIC & SIMPLE RECIPES 17
   1. Keto Mac & Cheese 18
   2. Mediterranean Salmon with Asparagus 20
BREAK FAST & EGGS 23
   3. Berry Hemp Seed Breakfast 24
   4. Morning Chia Pudding 26
   5. Broccoli, Egg & Pancetta Gratin 28
SALADS & SOUPS 31
   6. Picled Pepper Salad with Grilled Steak 32
   7. Parma Ham & Egg Salad 34
   8. Chicken Salad with Gorgonzola Cheese 36
   9. Cream of Roasted Jalapeño Soup 38
POULTRY 41
   10. Baked Chicken Legs with Tomato Sauce 42
   11. Coconut Chicken with Asparagus Sauce 44
   12. Citrus Chicken with Spinach & Pine Nuts 46
   13. Easy Pulled Chicken with Avocado 48
   14. Mustard Chicken with Rosemary 50
   15. Chicken Balls with Spaghetti Squash 52
BEEF & LAMB 55
   16. Asian-Style Creamy Beef 56
   17. Beef Hot Dogs in Bacon Wraps 58

18. Jerked Beef Stew 60

19. Coconut-Olive Beef with Mushrooms 62

20. Cilantro Beef Curry with Cauliflower 64

21. Beef Fajitas with Colorful Bell Peppers 66

FISH & SEAFOOD 69

22. Parmesan Shrimp Scampi Pizza 70

23. Spiralized Zucchini with Garlic Shrimp 72

VEGETABLE SIDES & DAIRY 75

24. Tofu & Parsnip Spaghetti a la "Bolognese" 76

25. Vegetable Keto Pasta Gratin 78

26. Balsamic Zoodles with Broccoli & Peppers 80

27. Mushroom & Zucchini with Spinach Dip 82

VEGAN 85

28. Fennel & Celeriac with Chili Tomato Sauce 86

29. Poppy Seed Coleslaw 88

SNACKS & APPETIZERS 91

30. Cheesy Bacon Bites 92

31. Cheesy Green Bean & Bacon Roast 94

32. Parsley Cauliflower & Bacon Stir-Fry 96

33. Artichoke & Bacon Gratin with Cauli Rice 98

34. Oregano Parsnip Mash with Ham 100

35. Pancetta-Wrapped Strawberries 102

36. Spicy Cauliflower Falafel 104

SMOOTHIES & BEVERAGES 107

37. Almond-Raspberry Smoothie 108

SWEETS & DESSERTS 111

38. Chocolate Avocado Truffles 112

39. Coconut Fat Bombs...114

40. Maple-Berry Fat Bombs...116

41. Peanut Butter Fat Bombs...118

42. Cheesy Fat Bombs with Brewed Coffee...120

43. Strawberry Trifle with Hazelnuts..122

44. No-Bake Peanut Butter Cookies..124

45. Chorizo & Cabbage Bake...126

KETO SMALL APPLIANCE RECIPES...129

46. Slow Cooker Turnip Soup with Sour Cream...................................130

47. Instant Pot Chicken Lazone...132

48. Instant Pot No Bean Chicken Chili..134

49. Instant Pot Chicken Soup..136

50. Sous Vide Buffalo Chicken Wings...138

MEASUREMENTS & CONVERSIONS...140

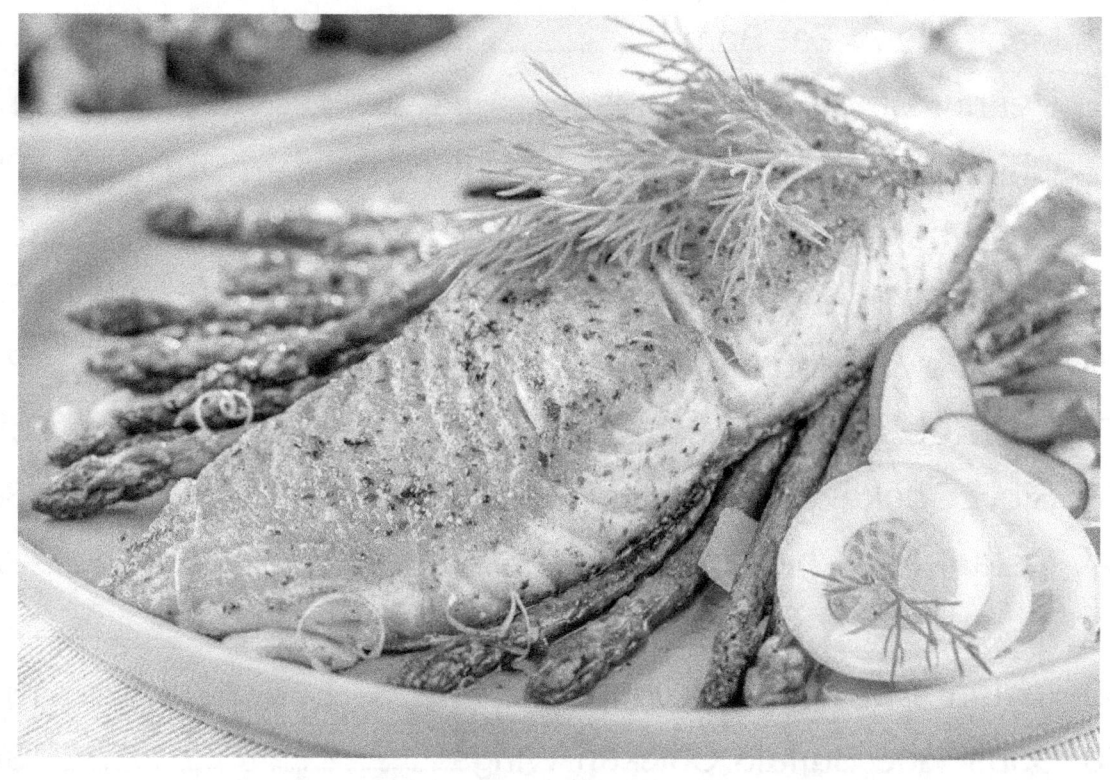

INTRODUCTION

It's widely-spread knowledge that our bodies are designed to run primarily on carbs. We use them to provide our bodies with the energy required to boost our state, exercise, or just normal body functioning. However, most people are clueless about the fact that carbs are not the only source of fuel our bodies can use. Just like they can run on carbs, our bodies can also use fat sources. When we ditch the carbs and focus on providing our bodies with more fat, we are embarking on the ketogenic train.

The ketogenic diet is not just another fad diet. It has been around since 1920 and has resulted in outstanding results and amazingly successful stories. If you are new to the keto world and have no idea what I am talking about, let me simplify this for you.

For you to truly understand what the keto diet is all about and why you should start it as soon as you can, let me first explain what happens to your body after consuming a carb-loaded meal.

Imagine you have just swallowed a giant bowl of spaghetti. Your tummy is full, your taste buds are satisfied, and your body is provided with more carbs than necessary. After consumption, your body immediately starts the process of digestion, during which your body will break down the consumed carbs into glucose, which is a source of energy your body depends on. So one might ask, "What is wrong with carbs?" For starters, there are some things: they raise the blood sugar, make your body work excessively to offset the effects of that sugar, and kindly storing it as another layer of fat, usually around the belly, but many times around the organs too. That's extremely dangerous. Sounds scary? I know.

By now, you've undoubtedly heard of the keto diet and the many people who have had success losing weight and keeping it off. But just what is a ketogenic diet, and how does it work to reach your weight loss goal.

The keto diet is a food plan that is high in fat and low in carbs. The human body uses carbohydrates as its primary fuel source; however, when fats replace carbs, the body enters a metabolic state known as "ketosis." During

ketosis, because of the lack of carbs, the body will burn stored fat as fuel, which can help you lose weight.

Not only can the keto diet promote weight loss, but it also comes with numerous health benefits:

- Management of diabetes
- Lower cholesterol
- Improved mental clarity
- Reduces the risk and symptoms of polycystic ovary syndrome (POS)
- Lower risk of some cancers
- Lower risk of cardiovascular disease

The keto diet requires a change in your wearing habits. It's easier to make these changes when you have your partner or other family members' active support. As a couple, you'll be able to encourage each other on those days that are more difficult than others for sticking to your food plan.

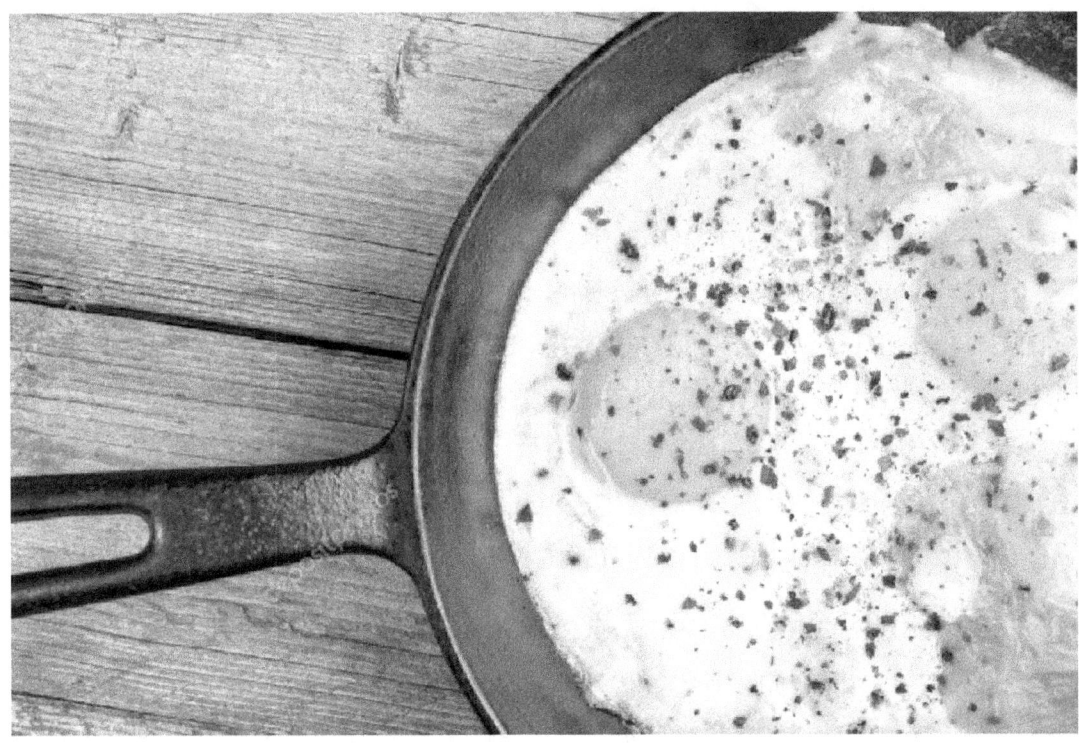

THE KETOSIS

Switching to high fat moderate protein cycle, your liver now has a new "fuel boss" - the fat. Once your liver begins preparing your body for the fuel change, the fat from the liver will start producing ketones – hence the name Ketogenic. What glucose is for the carbs, the ketones are for the fat, meaning they are the tiny molecules created once the fat is broken down to be used as energy. The switch from glucose to ketones is something that has pushed many people away from this diet. Some people consider this to be a dangerous process, but the truth is, your body will run just as efficiently on ketones as it does on glucose.

Once your body shifts to using ketones as fuel, you are in the state of ketosis. Ketosis is a metabolic process that may be interpreted as a little 'shock' to your body. However, this is far from dangerous. Every change in life requires adaptation, and so does this. This adaptation process is not set in stone, and every person goes through ketosis differently. However, for most people, it takes around 2 weeks to adapt to the new lifestyle fully.

Note! This is all biological and completely healthy. You have spent your whole life packing your body with glucose; naturally, you need time to adapt to the new dietary change.

Foods Allowed On the Keto Diet

Plan your meals and snacks around the following foods:

- Eggs
- Meats, including beef, pork, chicken, and veal
- Fish, including fish high in fat such as mackerel, trout, and salmon
- Cheeses
- Nuts and seeds, including nut and seed butter

- Cream and butter
- Avocadoes
- Healthy oils, such as olive, avocado, and coconut oils
- Low-carb vegetables, such as peppers, onions, tomatoes, and green vegetables
- Herbs and spices, including salt and pepper

To be sure you're getting enough of the right nutrients, eat a wide variety of meats, vegetables, seeds, and nuts on the allowed food list.

Foods Restricted On the Keto Diet

These are the foods that are restricted on a ketogenic food plan:

- Grains and starches, such as bread, pasta, cereal, and rice
- Carrots, potatoes, yams, sweet potatoes, and parsnips
- Beans and legumes, including chickpeas, lentils, and peas
- Fruit, except for small quantities of berries
- Sugar in any form, including foods that contain fructose
- Processed diet foods and Alcohol
- Condiments that contain sugar
- Unhealthy fats, such as processed vegetable oils and mayonnaise
- Alcohol

Getting Started with Your Keto Diet

Before starting the keto diet, take some time researching the foods on the allowed list and those restricted foods. Plan your meals ahead of time and shop accordingly, filling your kitchen with keto-friendly foods.

Healthy snacks

To make it easier to stick to the keto diet, it's important to have healthy snacks. If you're on the keto diet with your partner, have keto-approved snacks on hand that you both enjoy. Approved snacks include:

- Hard-boiled eggs, cheese, and olives
- A handful of nuts and seeds
- Celery and red pepper sticks with guacamole and salsa
- No-sugar plain yogurt mixed with berries

Intermittent Fasting and the Keto Diet

Intermittent fasting is all about restricting the number of calories you consume within a period so that you put your body into a "fasted" state. When this happens, the body's insulin levels will start to lower, which increases the fat burning process.

The Benefits of Intermittent Fasting Include:

- Weight loss
- Improved mental clarity
- Management and reducing the risk of type 2 diabetes
- Lower risk of cardiovascular disease
- Lower risk of some cancers

The most common fasting method is to fast each day for 14 to 16 hours, restricting the time you eat to a "window" of 8 to 10 hours. During the eating window, you should be eating at least 2 to 3 healthy keto meals. An excellent way to approach intermittent fasting is eating your last meal by 8 pm on any day and not eating your first meal until midnight the next day.

Another intermittent fasting method includes the 5:2 rule, where you only eat 500 to 600 calories per day on two days of the week, eating a healthy keto diet for the other five days. Another fasting method is the eat-stop-eat plan, where you fast for 24 hours twice a week.

Both intermittent fasting and the keto diet put the body into a ketosis state to use up stored fat for energy. When you combine intermittent fasting with the keto diet, you may be able to put your body into ketosis faster than dieting alone. This can lead to faster and more efficient weight loss.

What to Expect On the Keto Diet & Keto "Flu"

During the first few days of starting the Keto, you may experience an increase in hunger, lack of energy, and problems sleeping. Some people may also experience nausea and digestive issues. These flu-like symptoms are known as the "keto flu." To alleviate these symptoms, consider doing a low-carb diet for a week slowly transitioning into the full keto diet. During the first month, always eat until you feel full without focusing on restricting calories. Ease into the food plan, so you're less likely to stop eating a ketogenic diet.

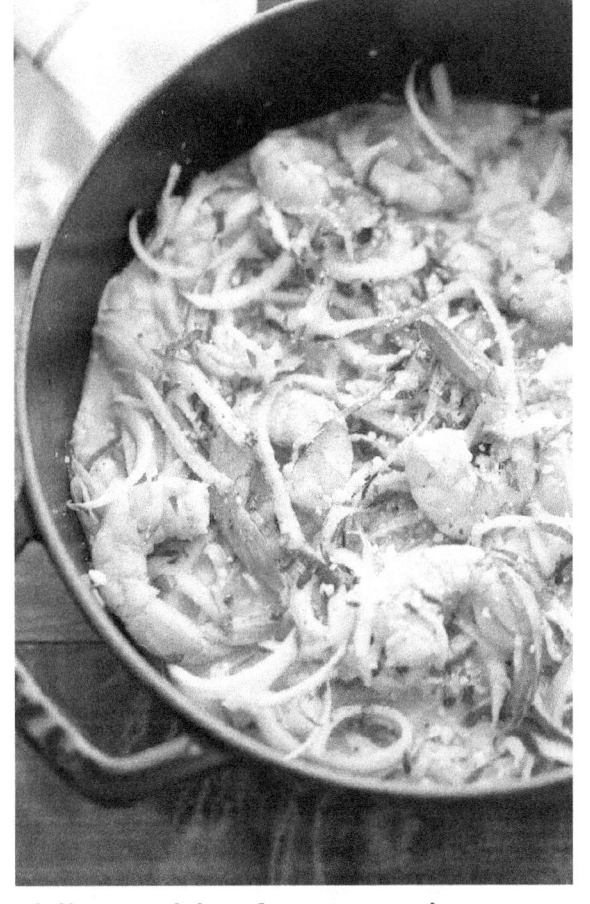

The keto diet changes the mineral and water balance of your body. Make sure that you're drinking more water each day. As well, taking a mineral supplement and adding a bit of extra salt to your diet can keep help maintain a healthy balance of minerals and water, helping to relieve any of the flu-like symptoms. For a mineral supplement, take 300 mg of magnesium and 1,000 mg of potassium.

DIET – THE NEW LIFESTYLE

The Benefits of Keto Diet

Even though it is still considered 'controversial,' the keto diet is the best dietary choice one can make. From weight loss to longevity, here are the benefits that following a ketogenic diet can bring to your life:

Loss of Appetite

You can't tame your cravings? Don't worry. While on ketosis, you won't feel exhausted or with a rumbling gut. The keto diet will help you say no to that second piece of cake. Once you train your body to run on fat and not on carbs, you will experience a drop in appetite that will work magic for your figure.

Weight Loss

Since the body is forced to produce only a small amount of glucose, it will lower insulin production. When that happens, your kidneys will start getting rid of the extra sodium, which will lead to weight loss.

HDL Cholesterol Increase and Drop in Blood Pressure

While consuming a diet high in fat and staying clear of harmful glucose, your body will experience a rise in good HDL cholesterol levels, which will, in turn, reduce the risk for many cardiovascular problems. Cutting back on carbs will also drop your blood pressure. The drop in blood pressure can prevent many health problems such as strokes or heart diseases.

Lower Risk of Diabetes

Although this probably goes without saying, it is essential to mention this one. When you ditch the carbs, your body is forced to lower the glucose productivity significantly, which leads to a lower risk of diabetes, including a reverse in the condition if you already have it.

Improved Brain Function

Many studies have shown that replacing carbohydrates with fat as an energy source leads to mental clarity and improved brain function. This is yet another reason why you should go Keto.

Should You Try the Keto Diet?

The keto diet can help you lose weight and keep it off. When you're eating nutritiously, exercising, and following a ketogenic food plan, you'll be joining the many other people around the world who have successfully lost weight.

Whether you're starting the keto diet on your own or as a couple, begin with the keto food plan basics to become familiar with the foods you can and can't eat. As you start to lose weight and learn how to customize your meals, the keto diet plan will become a natural part of your lifestyle, allowing you to maintain your health and weight loss.

BASIC & SIMPLE RECIPES

1. KETO MAC & CHEESE

Ingredients

For 4 servings

- 4 zucchinis, cut into rings or spiralized
- 2 tbsp butter, melted
- Salt and black pepper, to taste
- 1 cup heavy cream
- 1 cup cream cheese
- 1 tsp garlic paste

Directions

Total Time: approx. 20 minutes

1. Top the zucchinis with melted butter, salt, and pepper and toss to coat. Cook in a saucepan over medium heat for 5-6 minutes. Remove to a serving plate.
2. In the same pan, pour the heavy cream, garlic paste, and cream cheese and heat through, stirring frequently. Reduce heat to low and simmer for 2-3 minutes or until the sauce thickens. Adjust the seasoning. Coat the zucchinis in the cheese sauce and serve immediately.

Per serving:

- Cal 686
- Fat 72g
- Net Carbs 3.9g
- Protein 10g

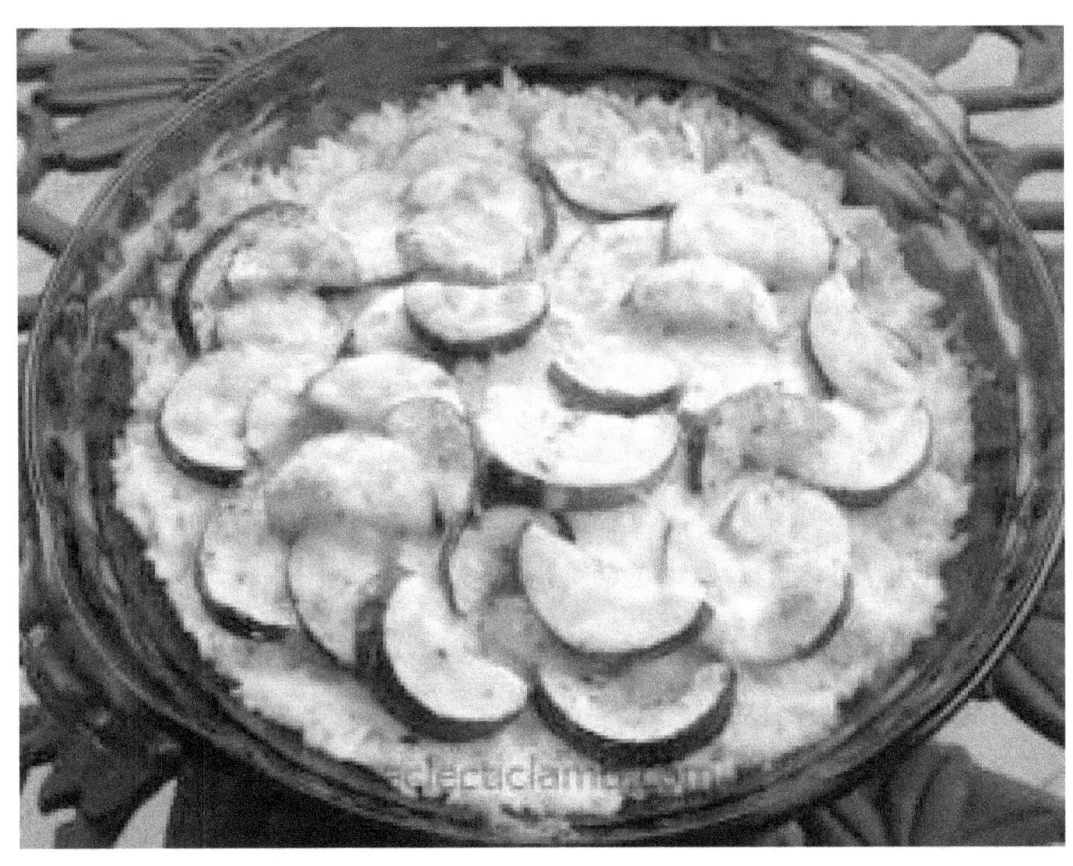

2. MEDITERRANEAN SALMON WITH ASPARAGUS

Ingredients

For 2 servings

- 2 tbsp olive oil
- ½ tsp dried dill
- ½ tsp garlic powder
- 2 salmon fillets
- ½ lemon, juiced
- ½ lb asparagus, trimmed
- ½ lemon, sliced thinly
- Salt and black pepper to taste

Directions

Total Time: approx. 30 minutes

1. Preheat the oven to 390 F. In a bowl, mix 1 tbsp of olive oil, dill, garlic powder, salt, and pepper.
2. Rub the mixture onto the salmon. Place the fish on a lined baking sheet.
3. Drizzle with lemon juice. Brush the asparagus with the remaining olive oil and season with salt and pepper.
4. Arrange asparagus around the salmon. Roast for 12-16 minutes, until the salmon fillets flake easily with a fork.
5. Serve topped with lemon slices.

Per serving:

- Cal 381
- Fat 25g
- Net Carbs 2.3g
- Protein 37g

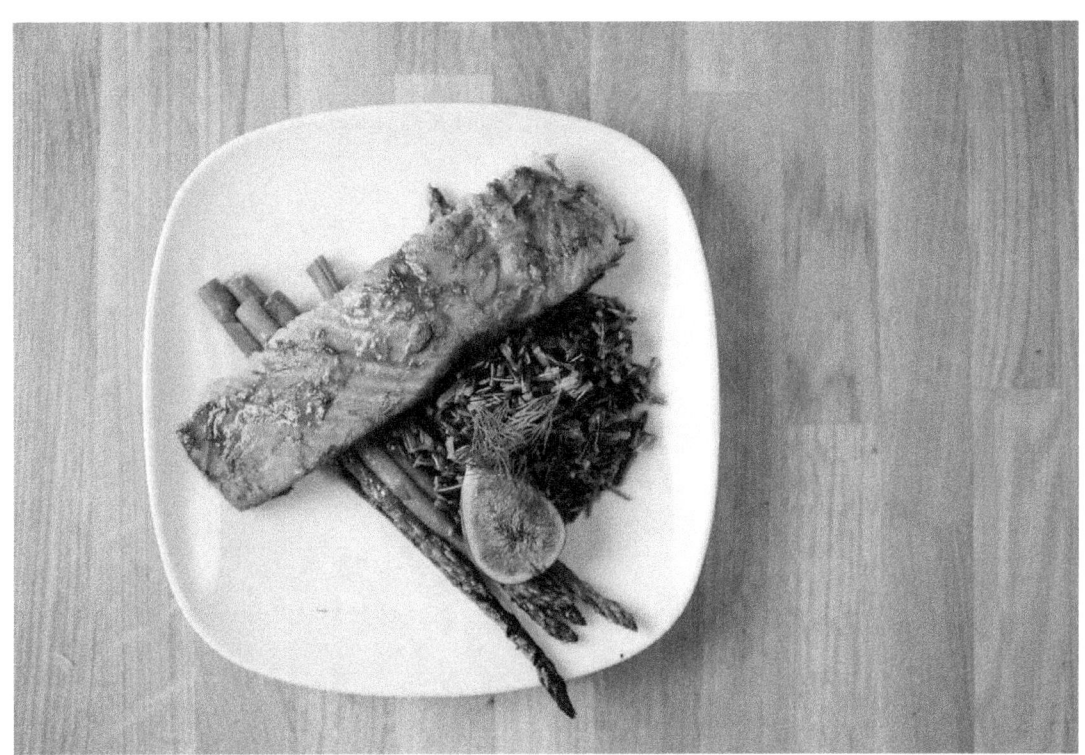

BREAK FAST & EGGS

3. BERRY HEMP SEED BREAKFAST

Ingredients

For 2 servings

- 1 cup berry medley
- 2 cups coconut milk
- ¼ tsp vanilla extract
- 4 oz heavy cream
- 2 tbsp hemp seeds
- 4 tsp liquid stevia
- 1 tbsp chopped pitted dates

Directions

Total Time: approx. 10 min + cooling time

1   Mash the berries with a fork until pureed in a medium bowl.

2   Pour in the coconut milk, heavy cream, hemp seeds, vanilla, and liquid stevia.

3   Mix and refrigerate the pudding overnight. Spoon the pudding into serving glasses, top with dates, and serve.

Per serving:

- Cal 532
- Fat 42g
- Net Carbs 5.3g
- Protein 14g

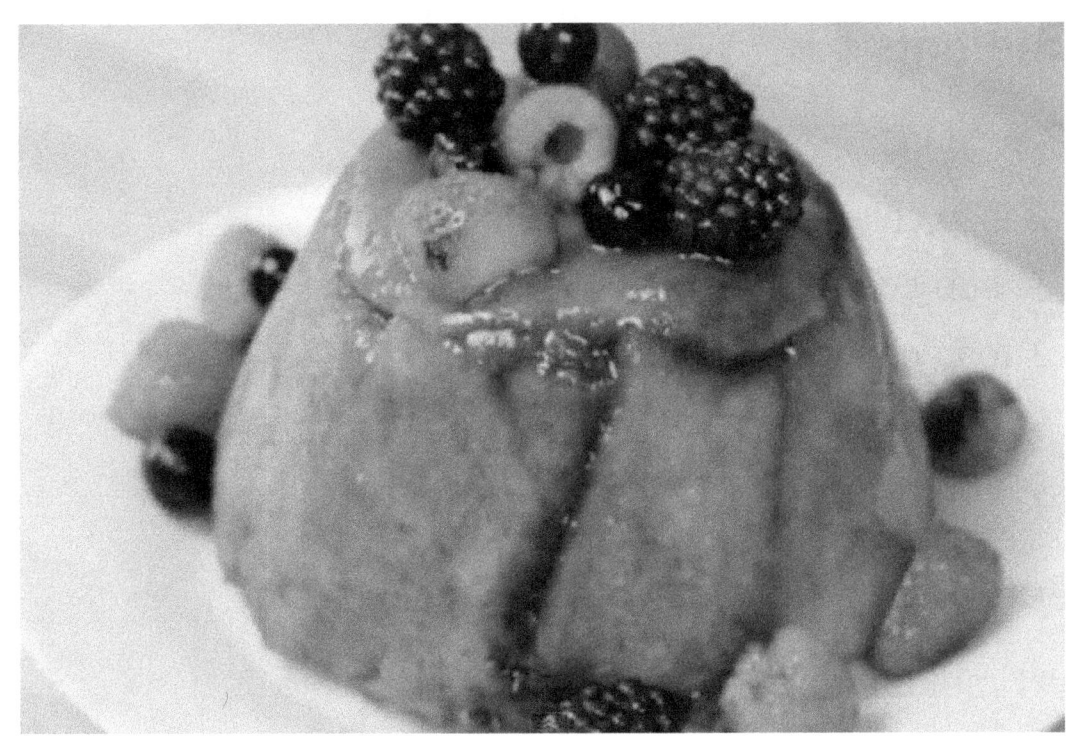

4. MORNING CHIA PUDDING

Ingredients

For 2 servings

- 2 tbsp chia seeds
- ¾ cup coconut milk
- 1 tbsp chopped walnuts
- ½ tsp vanilla extract
- ½ cup blueberries

Directions

Total Time: approx. 10 min + chilling time

1. Pour the coconut milk, vanilla, and half of the blueberries into a blender. Process the ingredients until the blueberries are incorporated into the liquid.
2. Mix in the chia seeds. Share the mixture into 2 jars, cover, and refrigerate for 4 hours to allow it to gel.
3. Garnish with the remaining blueberries and walnuts. Serve.

Per serving:

- Cal 299
- Net Carbs 6g
- Fat 19g
- Protein 9g

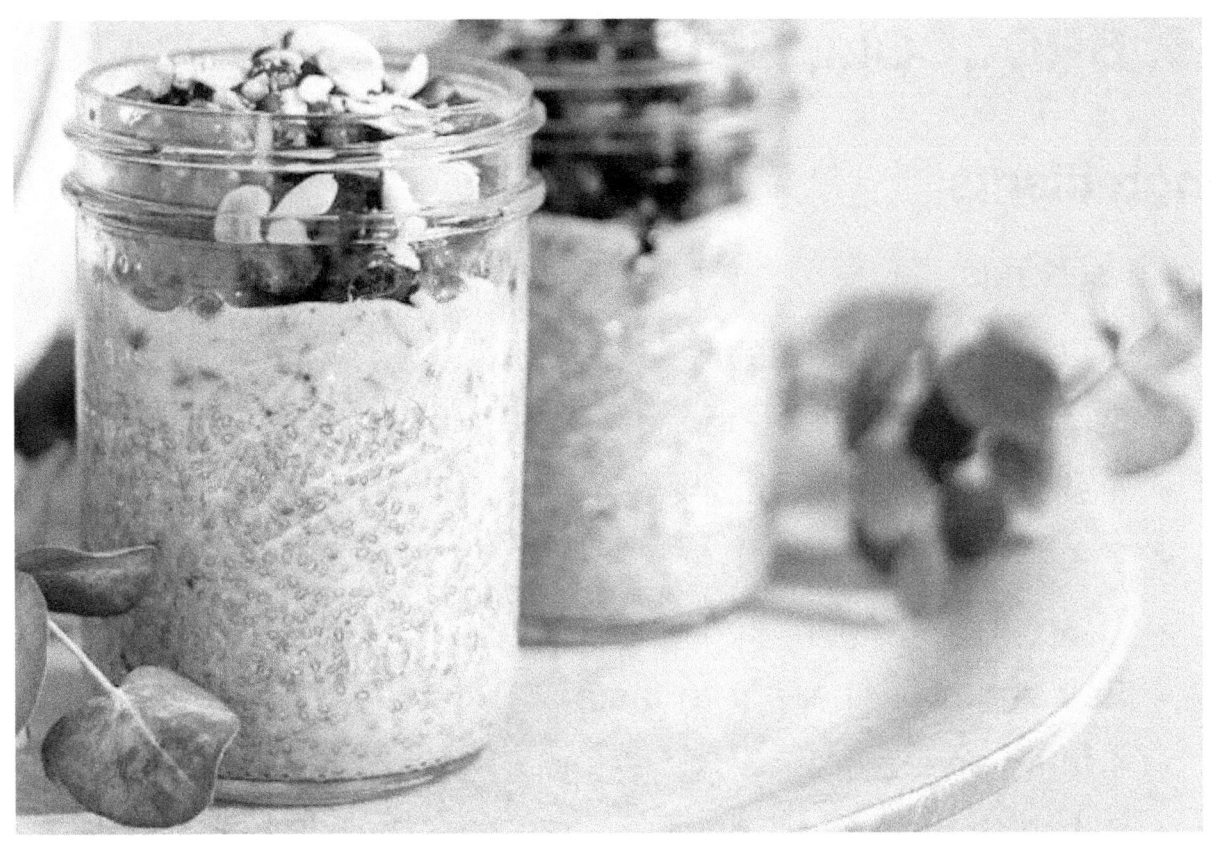

5. BROCCOLI, EGG & PANCETTA GRATIN

Ingredients

For 2 servings

- 10 oz broccoli florets
- 1 red bell pepper, chopped
- 4 slices pancetta, chopped
- 2 tsp olive oil
- 1 tsp dried oregano
- Salt and black pepper to taste
- 4 fresh eggs
- 4 tbsp Parmesan cheese

Directions

Total Time: approx. 30 minutes

1   Preheat oven to 420 F. Line a baking sheet with wax paper. Warm the olive oil in a pan over medium heat and stir-fry the pancetta for 3 minutes.

2   Place the broccoli, bell pepper, and pancetta on the baking sheet and toss to combine. Season with salt, oregano, and pepper.

3   Bake for 10 minutes until the vegetables have softened.

4   Remove, create 4 indentations, and crack an egg into each one. Sprinkle with Parmesan cheese.

5   Return to the oven and bake for 5-7 minutes or until the egg whites are firm and the cheese melts. Remove from

the oven and serve.

Per serving:

- Cal 464
- Fat 38g
- Net Carbs 4.2g
- Protein 24g

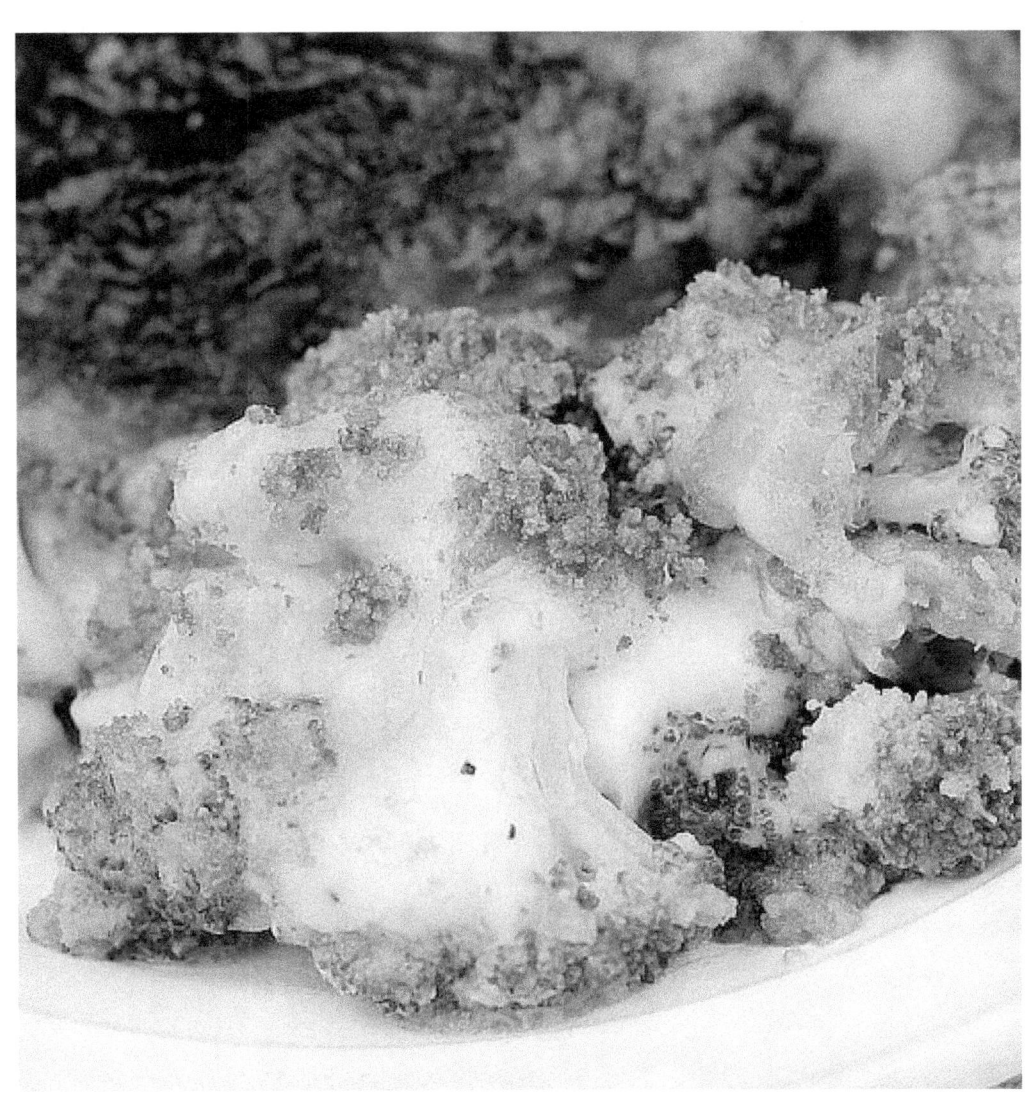

SALADS & SOUPS

6. PICLED PEPPER SALAD WITH GRILLED STEAK

Ingredients

For 2 servings

- ½ cup feta cheese, crumbled
- 1 lb skirt steak, sliced
- Salt and black pepper to taste
- 1 tsp olive oil
- 1 cup lettuce salad
- 1 cup arugula
- 3 pickled peppers, chopped
- tbsp red wine vinegar

Directions

Total Time: approx. 15 minutes

1 Preheat grill to high heat. Season the steak slices with salt and black pepper and drizzle with olive oil.

2 Grill the steaks on each side to the desired doneness, about 5-6 minutes. Remove to a bowl, cover, and leave to rest while you make the salad. Mix the lettuce salad and arugula, pickled peppers, and vinegar in a salad bowl.

3 Add the beef and sprinkle with feta cheese.

Per serving:

- Cal 633
- Fat 34g

- Net Carbs 4.7g
- Protein 72g

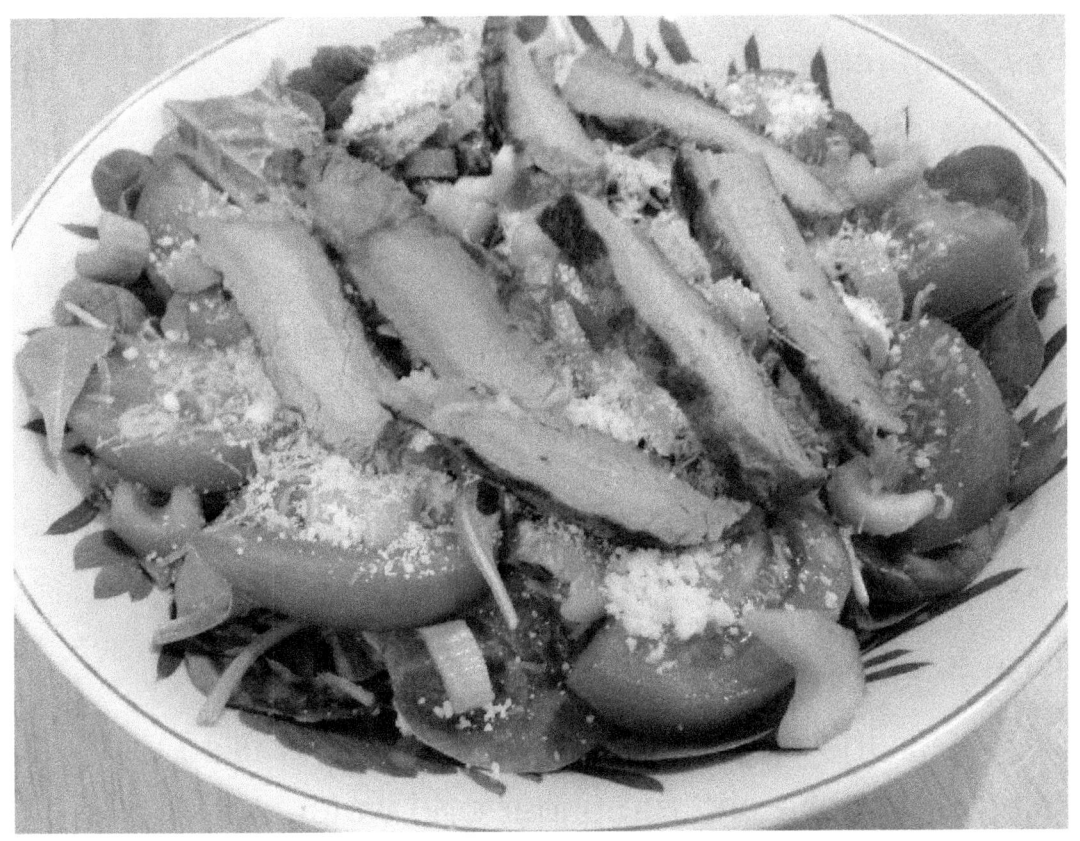

7. PARMA HAM & EGG SALAD

Ingredients

For 4 servings

- 8 eggs
- 1 /3 cup mayonnaise
- 1 tbsp minced onion
- ½ tsp mustard
- 1 ½ tsp lime juice
- Salt and black pepper, to taste
- 10 lettuce leaves
- 4 Parma ham slices

Directions

Total Time: approx. 20 minutes

1. Boil the eggs for 10 minutes in a pot filled with salted water. Remove and run under cold water.
2. Then peel and chop. Transfer to a mixing bowl together with the mayonnaise, mustard, black pepper, lime juice, onion, and salt.
3. Top with lettuce leaves and ham slices to serve.

Per serving:

- Cal 723
- Fat 53g
- Net Carbs 5.6g

- Protein 47g

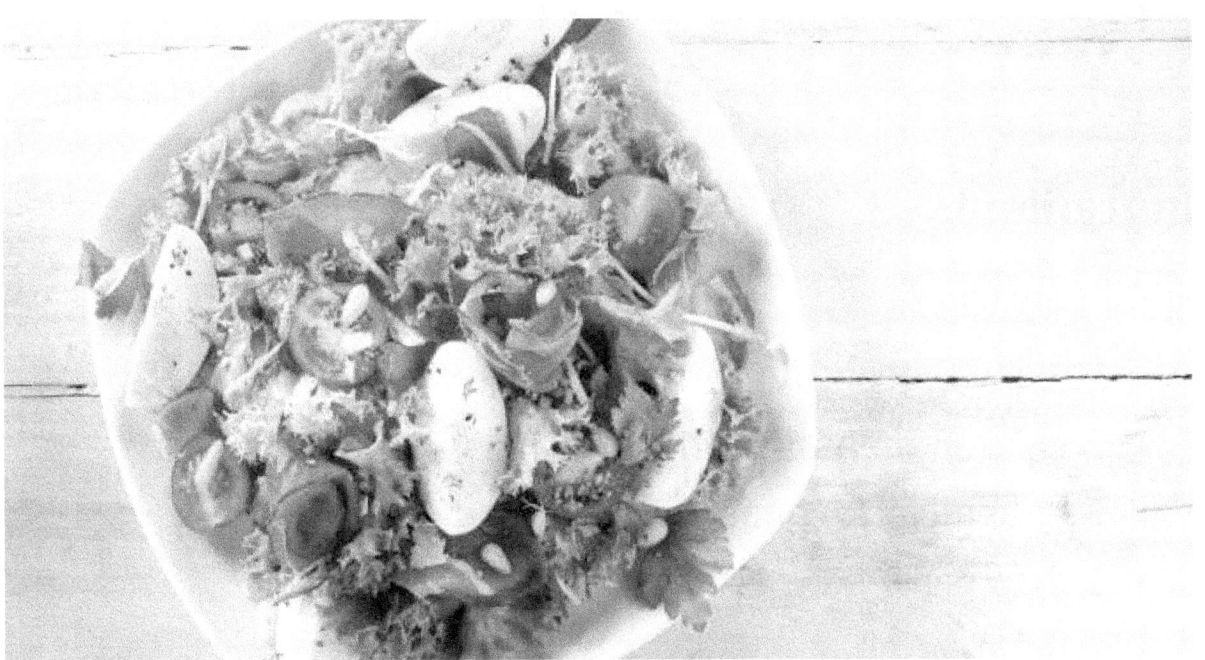

8. CHICKEN SALAD WITH GORGONZOLA CHEESE

Ingredients

For 2 servings

- ½ cup gorgonzola cheese, crumbled
- 1 chicken breast, boneless, skinless, flattened
- Salt and black pepper to taste
- 1 tbsp garlic powder
- 2 tsp olive oil
- 1 cup arugula
- 1 tbsp red wine vinegar

Directions

Total Time: approx. 15 minutes

1. Rub the chicken with salt, black pepper, and garlic powder. Heat half of the olive oil in a pan over medium heat and fry the chicken for 4 minutes on both sides or until golden brown. Remove to a cutting board and let cool before slicing.

2. Toss the arugula with vinegar and the remaining olive oil; share the salads onto plates. Arrange the chicken slices on top and sprinkle with gorgonzola cheese.

Per serving:

- Cal 291
- Fat 24g

- Net Carbs 3.5g
- Protein 12g

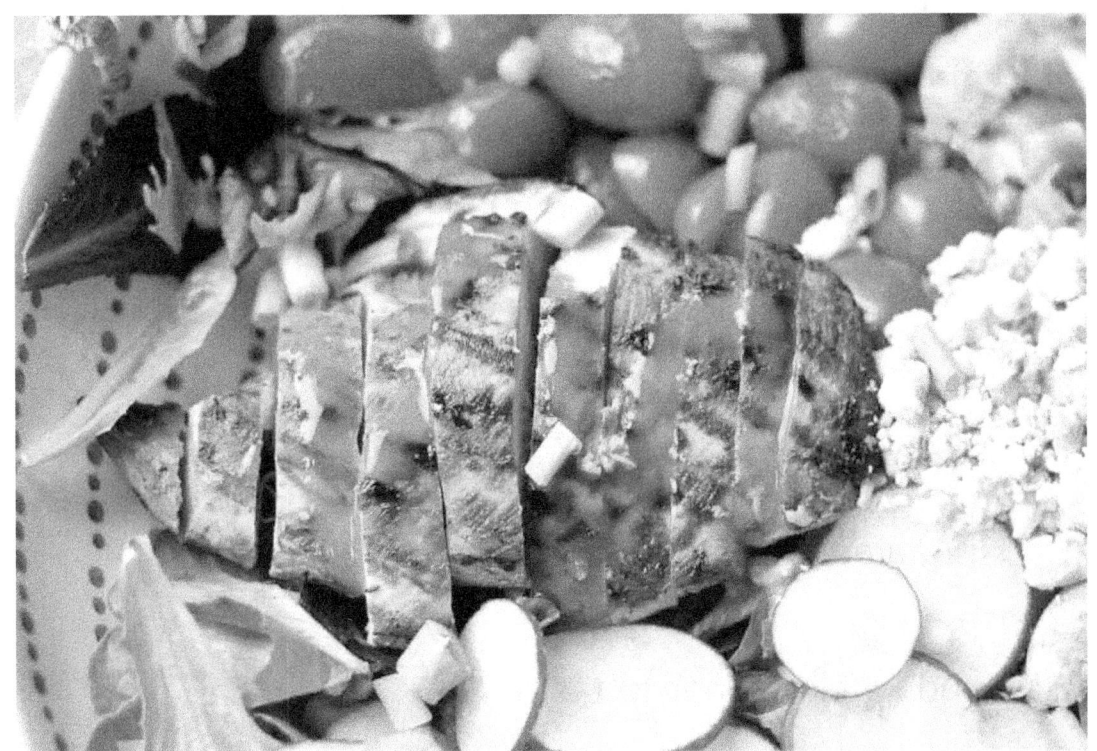

9. CREAM OF ROASTED JALAPEÑO SOUP

Ingredients

For 4 servings

- 2 tbsp melted butter
- 1 jalapeño pepper, halved
- 6 green bell peppers, halved
- 1 bulb garlic, halved, not peeled
- 6 tomatoes, halved
- 3 cups vegetable broth
- ½ cup heavy cream
- 3 tbsp grated Parmesan
- 2 tbsp chopped chives
- Salt and black pepper to taste

Directions

Total Time: approx. 45 min + cooling time

1   Preheat oven to 350 F. Arrange bell peppers, jalapeño pepper, and garlic on a baking pan and roast for 15 minutes.
2   Add in tomatoes and roast for 15 minutes. Let cool. Peel the skins and place them in a blender.
3   Add salt, pepper, butter, vegetable broth, and heavy cream; puree until smooth. Transfer to a pot over medium heat and cook for 3-4 minutes.
4   Serve into bowls sprinkled with Parmesan cheese and chives.

Per serving:

- Cal 191
- Net Carbs 8.7g
- Fat 9g
- Protein 5.3g

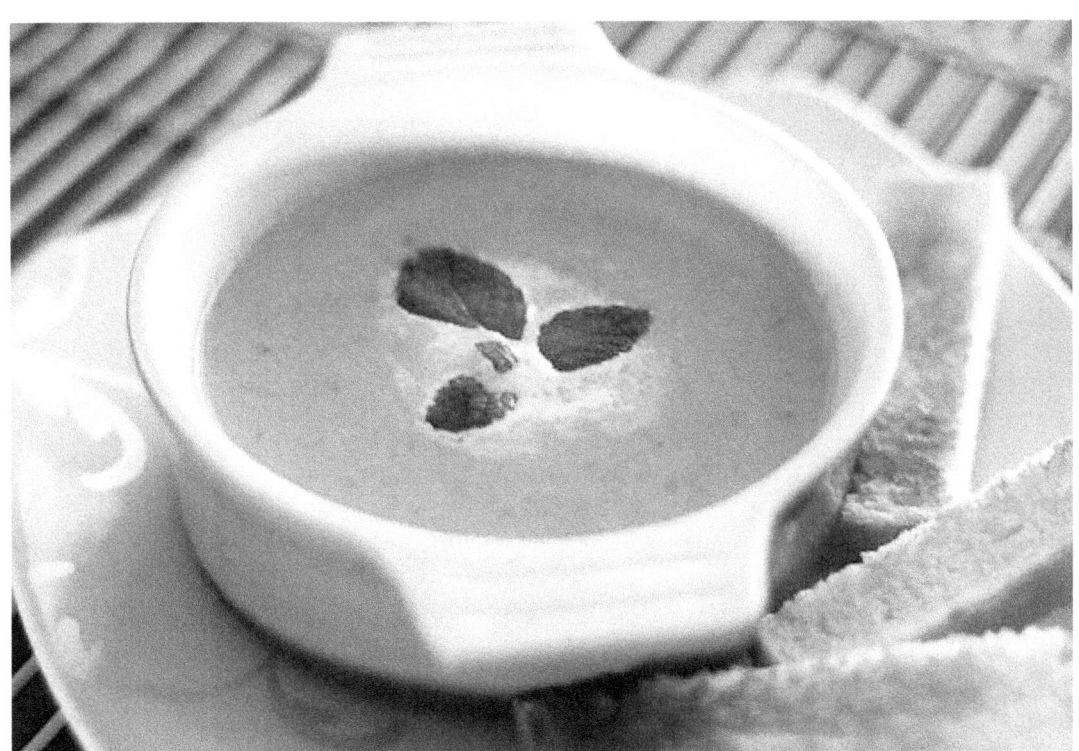

POULTRY

10. BAKED CHICKEN LEGS WITH TOMATO SAUCE

Ingredients

For 4 servings

- 1 (28 oz) can sugar- free tomato sauce
- 2 green bell peppers, cut into chunks
- 2 tbsp olive oil
- 1 lb chicken legs
- 2 green onions, chopped
- 1 parsnip, chopped
- 1 carrot, chopped
- 2 garlic cloves, minced
- ¼ cup coconut flour
- 1 cup chicken broth
- 2 tbsp Italian seasoning
- Salt and black pepper to taste

Directions

Total Time: approx. 1 hour 35 minutes

1   Season the legs with salt and black pepper. Heat the oil in a large skillet over medium heat and fry the chicken until brown on both sides for 10 minutes.

2   Remove to a baking dish. In the same pan, sauté the green onions, parsnip, bell peppers, carrot, and garlic for 10 minutes with continuous stirring.

3   In a bowl, evenly combine the broth, coconut flour, tomato sauce, and Italian seasoning together, and pour it over the vegetables in the pan.

4   Stir and cook to thicken for 4 minutes. Pour the mixture over the chicken in the baking dish, and bake in the oven for 1 hour at 390 F. Serve warm.

Per serving:

- Cal 345
- Fat 18g
- Net Carbs 9.5g
- Protein 25g

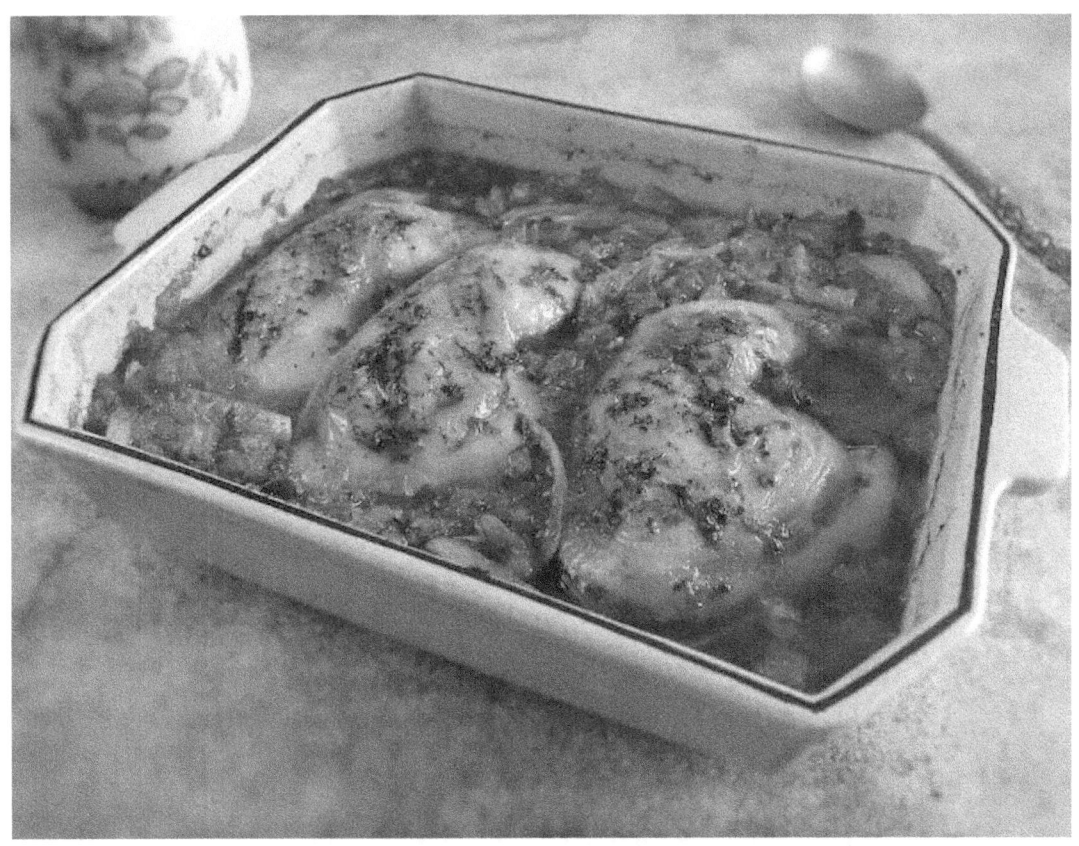

11. COCONUT CHICKEN WITH ASPARAGUS SAUCE

Ingredients

For 4 servings

- 1 tbsp butter
- 1 lb chicken thighs
- 2 tbsp coconut oil
- 2 tbsp coconut flour
- 2 cups asparagus, chopped
- 1 tsp oregano
- 1 cup heavy cream
- 1 cup chicken broth

Directions

Total Time: approx. 30 minutes

1   Melt the coconut oil in a skillet over medium heat. Brown the chicken on all sides, about 6-8 minutes. Set aside.

2   Melt the butter in the skillet and whisk in the flour and oregano.

3   Stir in heavy cream and chicken broth and bring to a boil.

4   Add the asparagus and cook for 10 minutes until tender. Transfer to a food processor and pulse until smooth.

5   Return to the skillet and add the chicken; cook for an additional 5 minutes and serve.

Per serving:

- Cal 451
- Fat 37g
- Net Carbs 3.2g
- Protein 18g

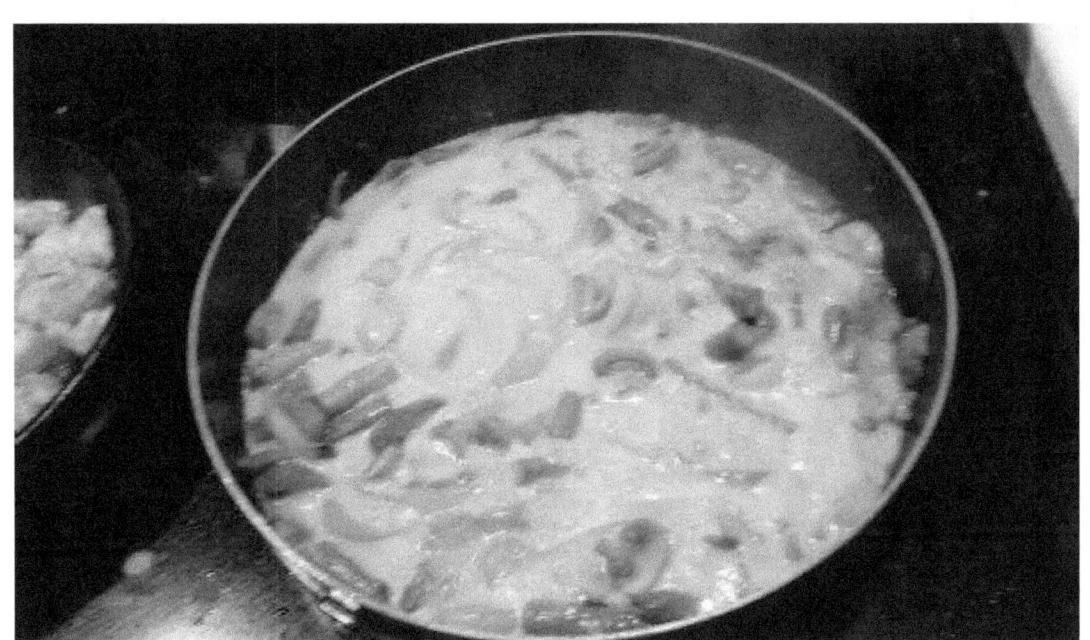

12. CITRUS CHICKEN WITH SPINACH & PINE NUTS

Ingredients

For 2 servings

- 2 tbsp olive oil
- 1 lb chicken thighs
- Salt and black pepper to serve
- 1 tbsp lemon juice
- 1 tsp lemon zest
- 1 tbsp oregano, chopped
- 1 garlic clove, minced
- 1 cup spinach
- 2 tbsp pine nuts

Directions

Total Time: approx. 20 min + chilling time

1   In a bowl, combine all ingredients, except olive oil, spinach, and pine nuts. Place in the fridge for 1 hour.

2   Warm the olive oil in a skillet over medium heat. Remove the chicken from the marinade, drain, and add to the pan.

3   Cook until crispy, about 7 minutes per side. Pour in the marinade and the spinach and cook for 4-5 minutes until the spinach wilts.

4   Serve sprinkled with pine nuts.

Per serving:

- Cal 465
- Fat 32g
- Net Carbs 3g
- Protein 29g

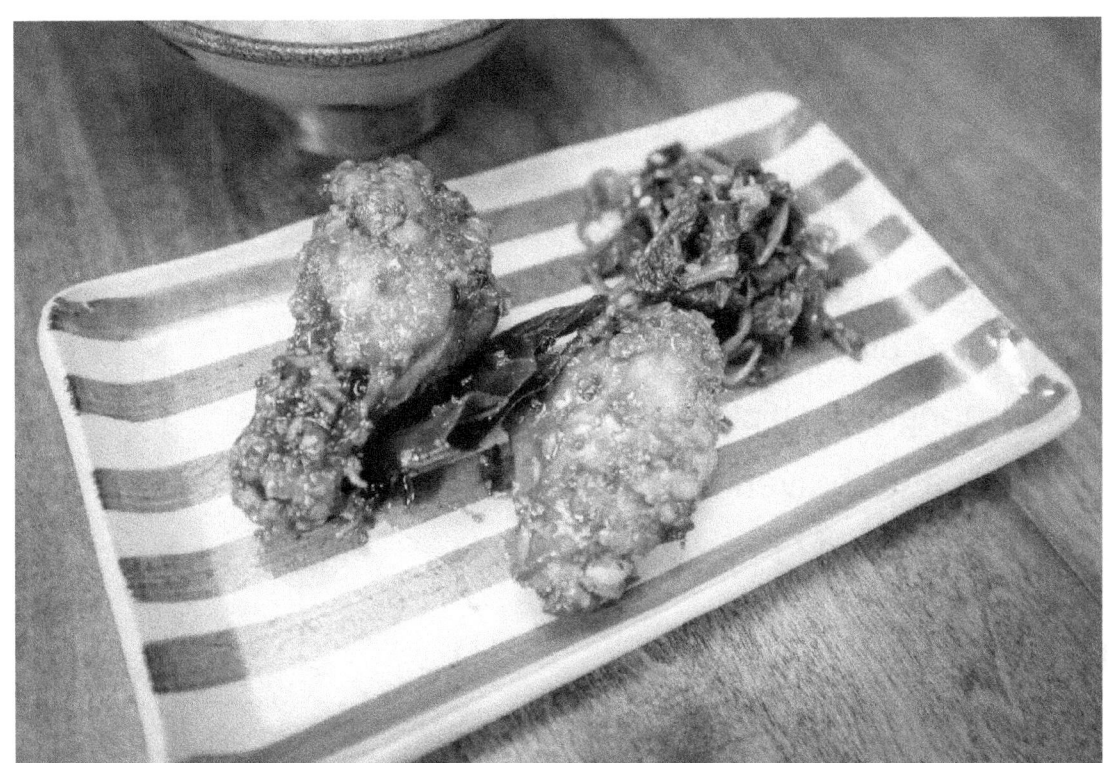

13. EASY PULLED CHICKEN WITH AVOCADO

Ingredients

For 4 servings

- 3 tbsp coconut oil
- 1 white onion, finely chopped
- ¼ cup chicken stock
- 3 tbsp tamari sauce
- 3 tbsp chili pepper
- 1 tbsp red wine vinegar
- Salt and black pepper to taste
- 2 lb boneless chicken thighs
- 1 avocado, halved and pitted
- ½ lemon, juiced

Directions

Total Time: approx. 2 hours 25 minutes

1   To a pot, add the onion, stock, coconut oil, tamari sauce, chili, vinegar, salt, and pepper and stir to combine.

2   Add in thighs, close the lid, and cook over low heat for 2 hours. Scoop avocado pulp into a bowl, add lemon juice, and mash the avocado into a puree; set aside.

3   When the chicken is ready, open the lid and use two forks to shred-it. Cook further for 15 minutes. Turn the heat off and mix in avocado. Serve warm.

Per serving:

- Cal 709
- Net Carbs 4g
- Fat 56g
- Protein 39g

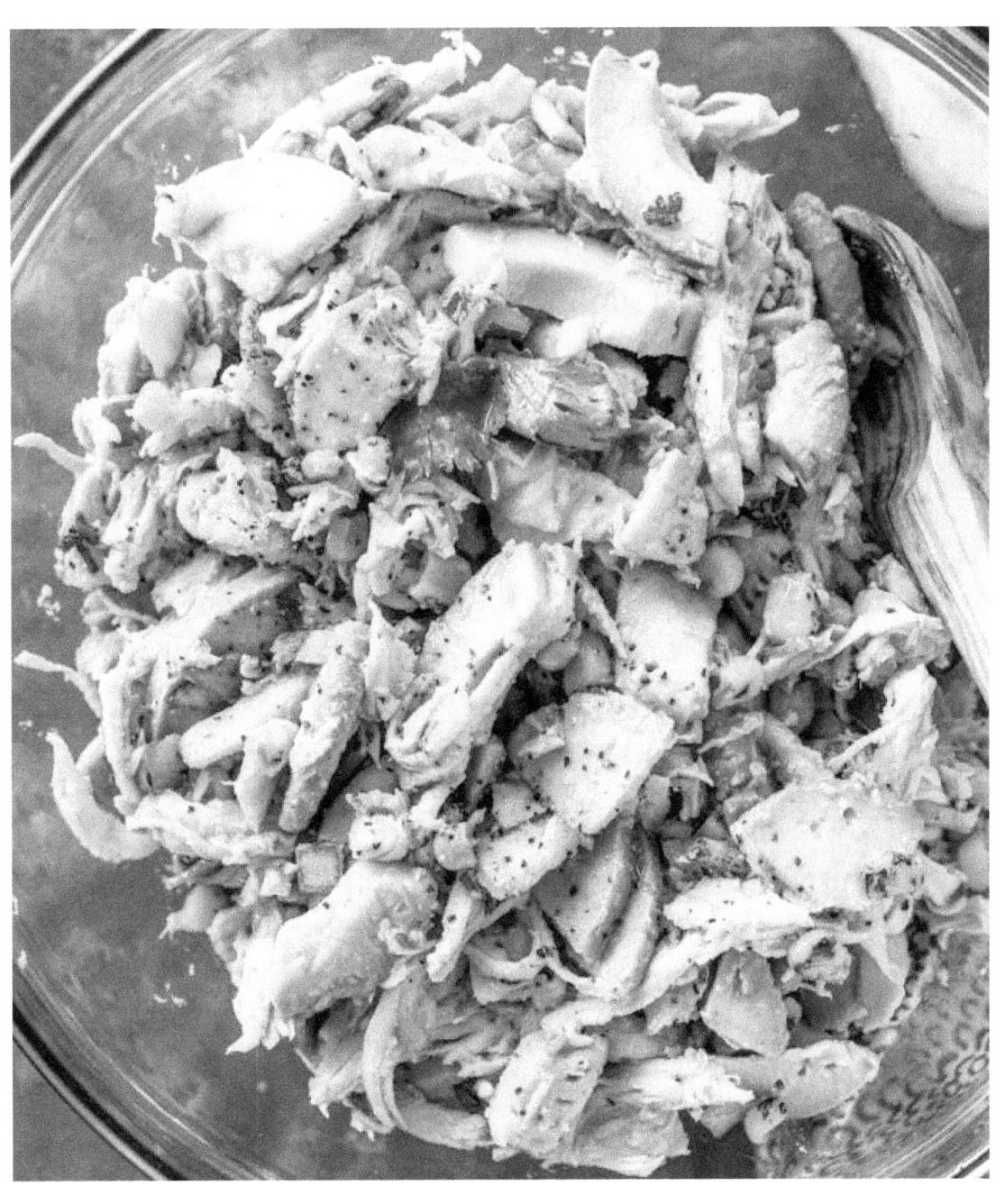

14. MUSTARD CHICKEN WITH ROSEMARY

Ingredients

For 4 servings

- 1 tbsp olive oil
- ½ cup chicken stock
- ½ cup onion, chopped
- 1 lb chicken thighs
- ¼ cup heavy cream
- 1 tbsp Dijon mustard
- 1 tsp rosemary, chopped
- Salt and black pepper to taste

Directions

Total Time: approx. 20 minutes

1. Warm the olive oil in a pan over medium heat. Season the chicken with salt and black pepper and cook for about 4 minutes per side; reserve.
2. Sauté the onion in the same pan for 3 minutes. Add the stock and simmer for 5 minutes.
3. Stir in mustard and heavy cream. Pour the sauce over the chicken and serve sprinkled with rosemary.

Per serving:

- Cal 515
- Fat 39g
- Net Carbs 5.2g

- Protein 32g

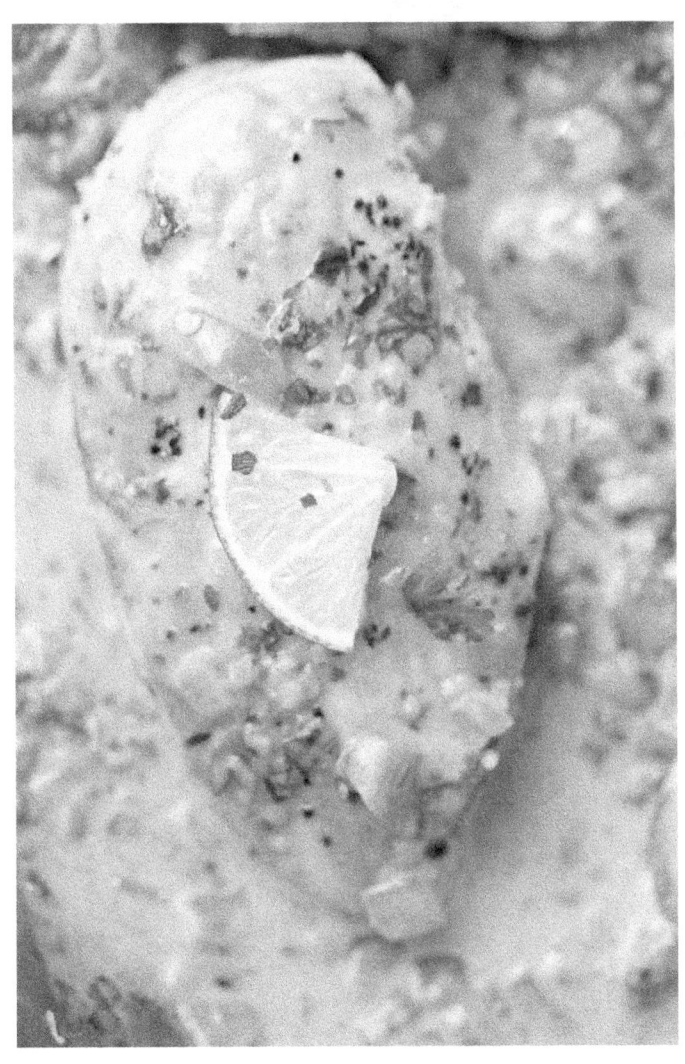

15. CHICKEN BALLS WITH SPAGHETTI SQUASH

Ingredients

For 4 servings

- ½ cup + 2 tbsp Pecorino cheese, grated
- 1 lb butternut squash, halved
- ½ lb ground chicken
- Salt to taste
- ½ cup pork rinds, crushed
- 1 garlic clove, minced
- 1 shallot, chopped
- 1 stalk celery, chopped
- 1 tbsp parsley, chopped
- 2 tbsp olive oil
- 1 red bell pepper, sliced
- 1 egg
- 1 cup sugar- free tomato sauce
- 1 tsp dried oregano
- 2 tbsp grated Parmesan cheese

Directions

Total Time: approx. 75 minutes

1 Preheat the oven to 450 F. Scoop the seeds out of the squash halves with a spoon. Sprinkle with salt and brush with 1 tbsp of olive oil. Place in a baking dish and roast for

30 minutes.

2   Scrape the pulp into strands. Remove the spaghetti strands to a bowl and toss with 2 tbsp of Pecorino cheese; set aside. Put the ground chicken in a bowl. Add in garlic, shallot, pork rinds, egg, oregano, and remaining Pecorino cheese; mix well. Mold out meatballs from the mixture and place them on a baking sheet. Bake the meatballs for just 10 minutes, but not done.

3   Place a pot over medium heat and warm the remaining olive oil. Stir in the tomato sauce, celery, red bell pepper, and salt to taste. Let the sauce cook on low-medium heat for 5 minutes.

4   Add in the meatballs. Continue cooking for 15 minutes. Spoon the meatballs with sauce over the spaghetti, sprinkle with Parmesan and parsley to serve.

Per serving:

- Cal 424
- Fat 28g
- Net Carbs 7.2g
- Protein 21g

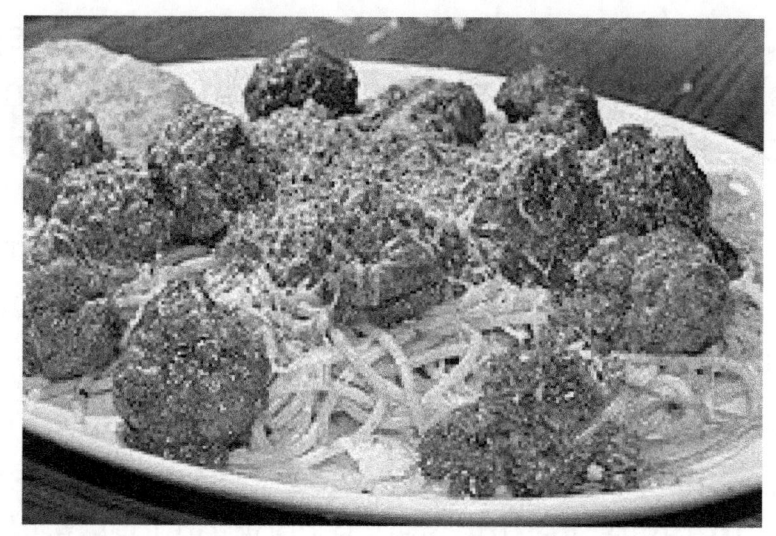

BEEF & LAMB

16. ASIAN-STYLE CREAMY BEEF

Ingredients

For 4 servings

- 4 large rib-eye steak
- 1 green bell pepper, sliced
- 1 red bell pepper, sliced
- 2 long red chilies, sliced
- 2 tbsp ghee
- 2 garlic cloves, minced
- ½ cup chopped brown onion
- 1 cup beef stock
- 1 cup coconut milk
- 1 tbsp Thai green curry paste
- 1 lime, juiced
- 2 tbsp chopped cilantro

Directions

Total Time: approx. 40 minutes

1. Warm the 1 tbsp of ghee in a pan over medium heat and cook the beef for 3 minutes on each side.

2. Remove to a plate. Add the remaining ghee to the skillet and sauté garlic and onion for 3 minutes.

3. Stir-fry in bell peppers and red chili until softened, 5 minutes. Pour in beef stock, coconut milk, curry paste, and lime juice. Let simmer for 4 minutes.

4   Put the beef back into the sauce. Cook for 10 minutes and transfer the pan to the oven. Cook further under the broiler for 5 minutes.

5   Garnish with cilantro and serve with cauliflower rice.

Per serving:

- Cal 638
- Net Carbs 2.6g
- Fat 35g
- Protein 69g

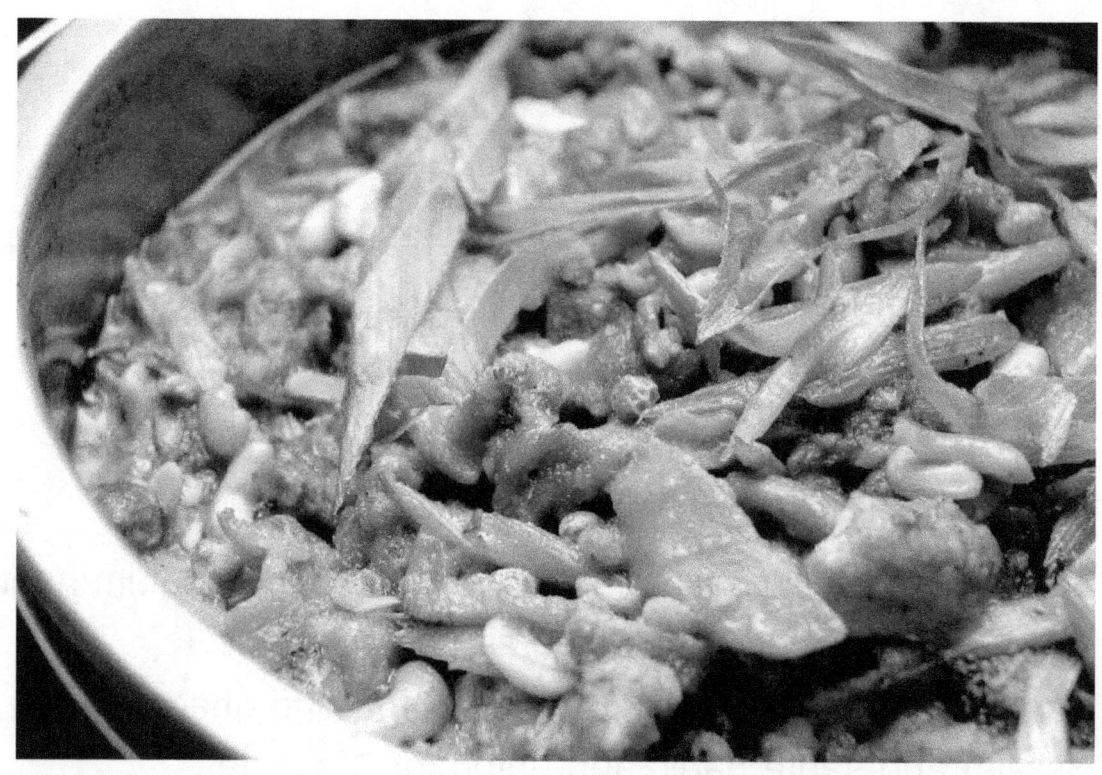

Questa foto di Autore sconosciuto è concesso in licenza da CC BY-ND

17. BEEF HOT DOGS IN BACON WRAPS

Ingredients

For 4 servings

- 16 bacon slices
- ½ cup grated Gruyere cheese
- 8 large beef hot dogs
- 1 tsp onion powder
- 1 tsp garlic powder
- Salt and black pepper to taste

Directions

Total Time: approx. 25 minutes

1. Preheat oven to 380 F. Cut a slit in the middle of each hot dog and stuff evenly with cheese.
2. Wrap each hot dog with 2 bacon slices and secure with toothpicks. Season with onion and garlic powders, salt, and pepper.
3. Place the hot dogs in the oven and slide in the cookie sheet beneath the rack to catch dripping grease.
4. Cook for 15 minutes until the bacon browns and crisps. Serve.

Per serving:

- Cal 763
- Net Carbs 4g
- Fat 61g

- Protein 42g

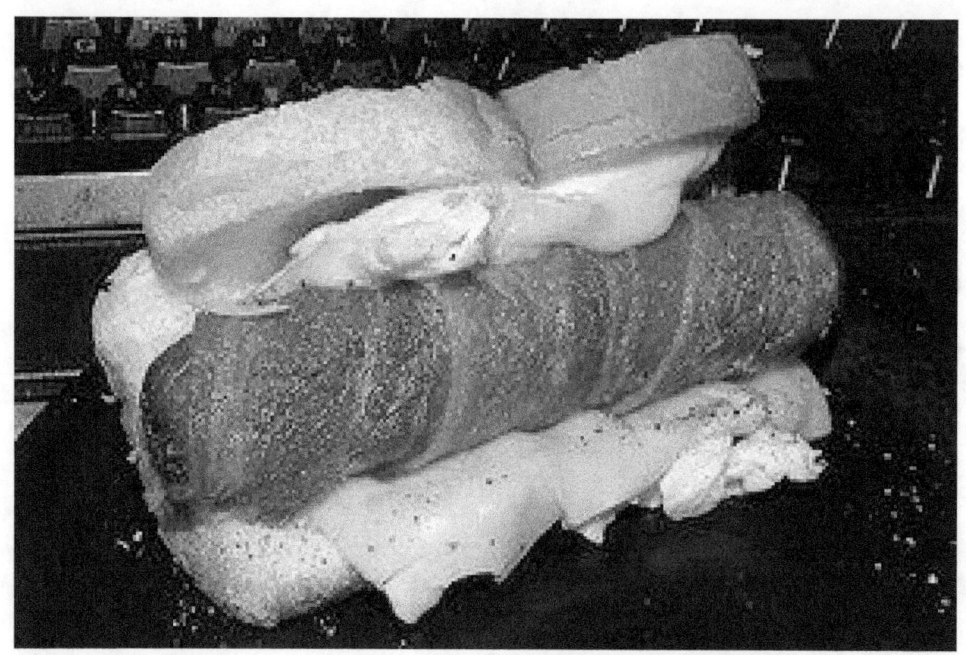

18. JERKED BEEF STEW

Ingredients

For 4 servings

- ½ scotch bonnet pepper, chopped
- 1 onion, chopped
- 2 tbsp olive oil
- 1 tsp ginger paste
- 1 tsp soy sauce
- 1 lb beef stew meat, cubed
- 1 red bell pepper, chopped
- 2 green chilies, chopped
- 1 cup tomatoes, chopped
- 1 tbsp fresh cilantro, chopped
- 1 garlic clove, minced
- ¼ cup vegetable broth
- Salt and black pepper to taste
- ¼ cup black olives, chopped
- 1 tsp jerk seasoning

Directions

Total Time: approx. 80 minutes

1 Brown the beef on all sides in warm olive oil over medium heat; remove and set aside.

2 Stir-fry in the red bell peppers, green chilies, jerk seasoning, garlic, scotch bonnet pepper, onion, ginger paste, and soy sauce, for about 5-6 minutes. Pour in the tomatoes

and broth, and cook for 1 hour.

3   Stir in the olives, adjust the seasonings and serve sprinkled with fresh cilantro.

Per serving:

- Cal 235
- Fat 13g
- Net Carbs 2.8g
- Protein 26g

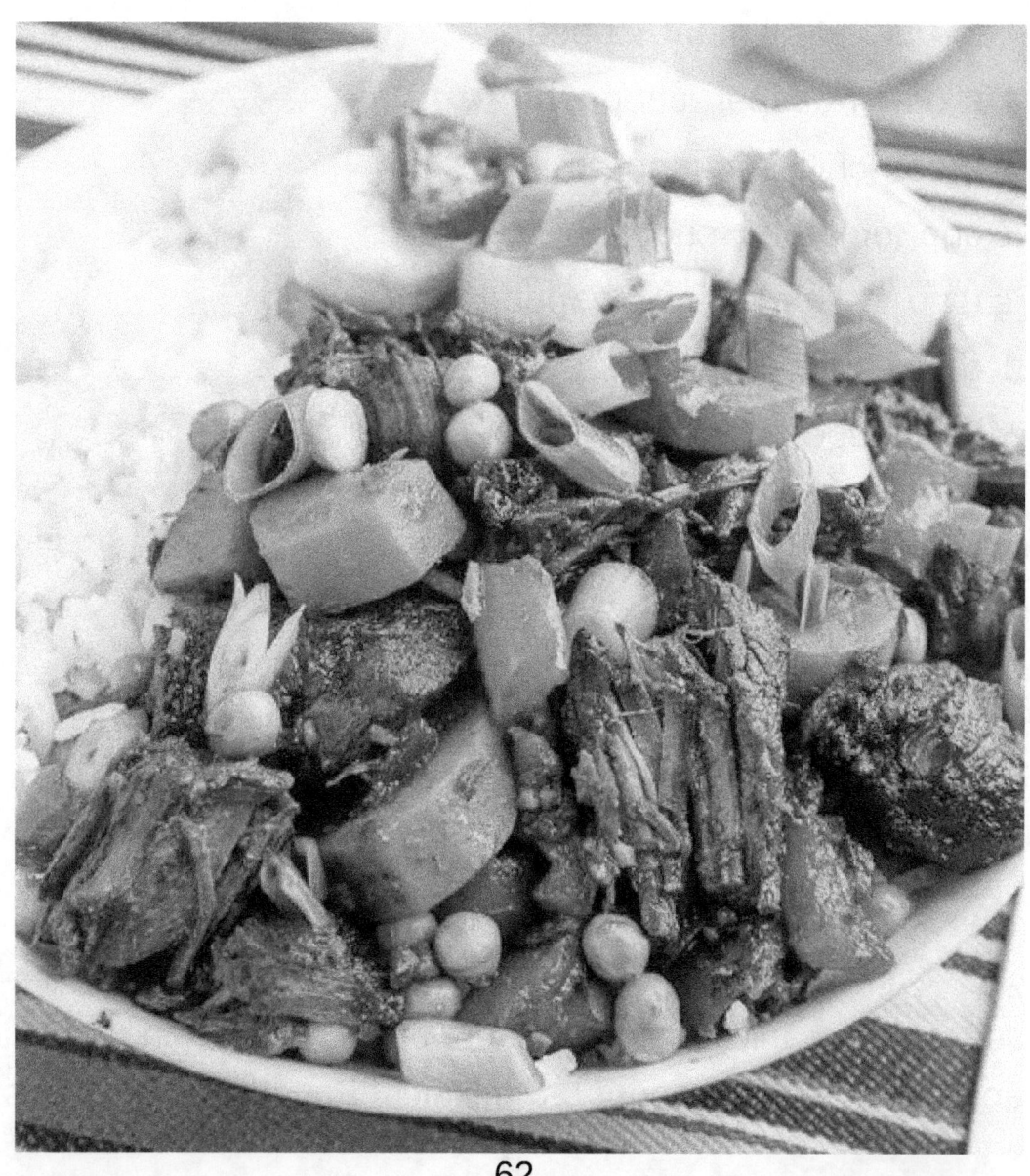

19. COCONUT-OLIVE BEEF WITH MUSHROOMS

Ingredients

For 4 servings

- ¼ cup button mushrooms, sliced
- 4 rib-eye steaks
- 3 tbsp butter
- 1 yellow onion, chopped
- 1/3 cup coconut milk
- 1 tbsp coconut cream
- 1/2 tsp dried thyme
- 2 tbsp chopped parsley
- 3 tbsp black olives, sliced

Directions

Total Time: approx. 30 minutes

1. Warm 2 tbsp butter in a deep skillet over medium heat.
2. Add and sauté the mushrooms for 4 minutes until tender.
3. Stir in onion and cook further for 3 minutes; set aside. Melt the remaining butter in the skillet and cook the beef for 10 minutes on both sides.
4. Pour mushrooms and onion back to the skillet and add milk, coconut cream, thyme, and 1 tbsp of parsley. Stir and simmer for 2 minutes.
5. Mix in black olives and turn the heat off.

6   Serve garnished with the remaining parsley.

Per serving:

- 3Cal 643
- Net Carbs 1.9g
- Fat 42g
- Protein 71g

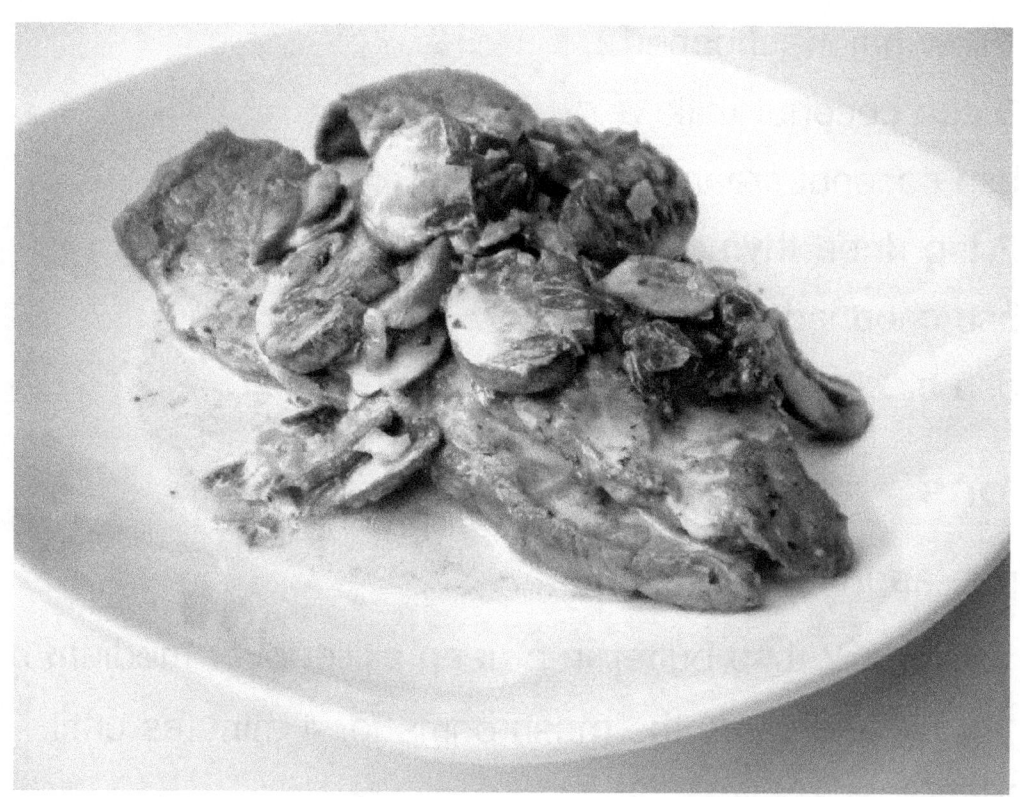

20. CILANTRO BEEF CURRY WITH CAULIFLOWER

Ingredients

For 4 servings

- 1 head cauliflower, cut into florets
- 1 tbsp olive oil
- ½ lb ground beef
- 1 garlic clove, minced
- 1 tsp turmeric
- 1 tbsp cilantro, chopped
- 1 tbsp ginger paste
- ½ tsp garam masala
- 5 oz canned whole tomatoes
- Salt and chili pepper to taste
- ¼ cup water

Directions

Total Time: approx. 30 minutes

1. Heat oil in a saucepan over medium heat, add the beef, garlic, ginger paste, and garam masala.
2. Cook for 5 minutes while breaking any lumps.
3. Stir in the tomatoes and cauliflower, season with salt, turmeric, and chili pepper, and cook covered for 6 minutes.
4. Add the water and bring to a boil over medium heat for 10 minutes or until the water has reduced by half.

5   Spoon the curry into serving bowls and serve sprinkled with cilantro.

Per serving:

- Cal 365
- Fat 32g
- Net Carbs 3.5g
- Protein 19g

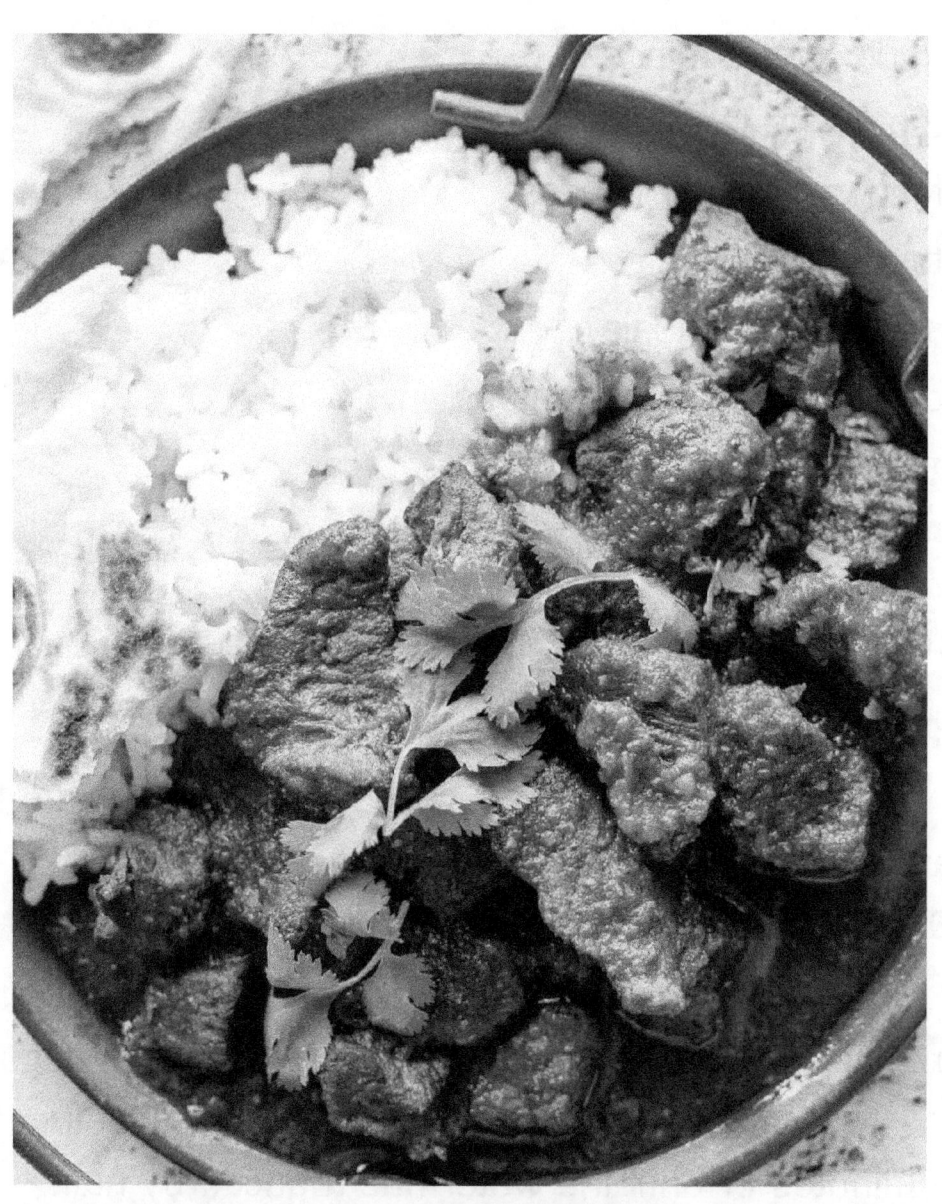

21. BEEF FAJITAS WITH COLORFUL BELL PEPPERS

Ingredients

For 4 servings

- 1 cup mixed bell peppers, chopped
- 2 tbsp olive oil
- 2 lb skirt steak, cut in halves
- 2 tbsp Cajun seasoning
- 2 large white onion, chopped
- ¼ cup cheddar cheese, grated
- 12 low carb tortillas

Directions

Total Time: approx. 35 min + cooling time

1. Rub the steak with Cajun seasoning and marinate in the fridge for one hour. Preheat grill to 400 F.
2. Cook the steak on the grill for 6 minutes on each side, flipping once until lightly browned. Remove from heat and cover with foil to sit for 10 minutes before slicing.
3. Heat the olive oil in a skillet over medium heat and sauté the onion and bell peppers for 5 minutes or until soft.
4. Cut steak against the grain into strips and share on the tortillas. Top with the veggies and cheese and serve.

Per serving:

- Cal 512

- Fat 32g
- Net Carbs 4g
- Protein 25g

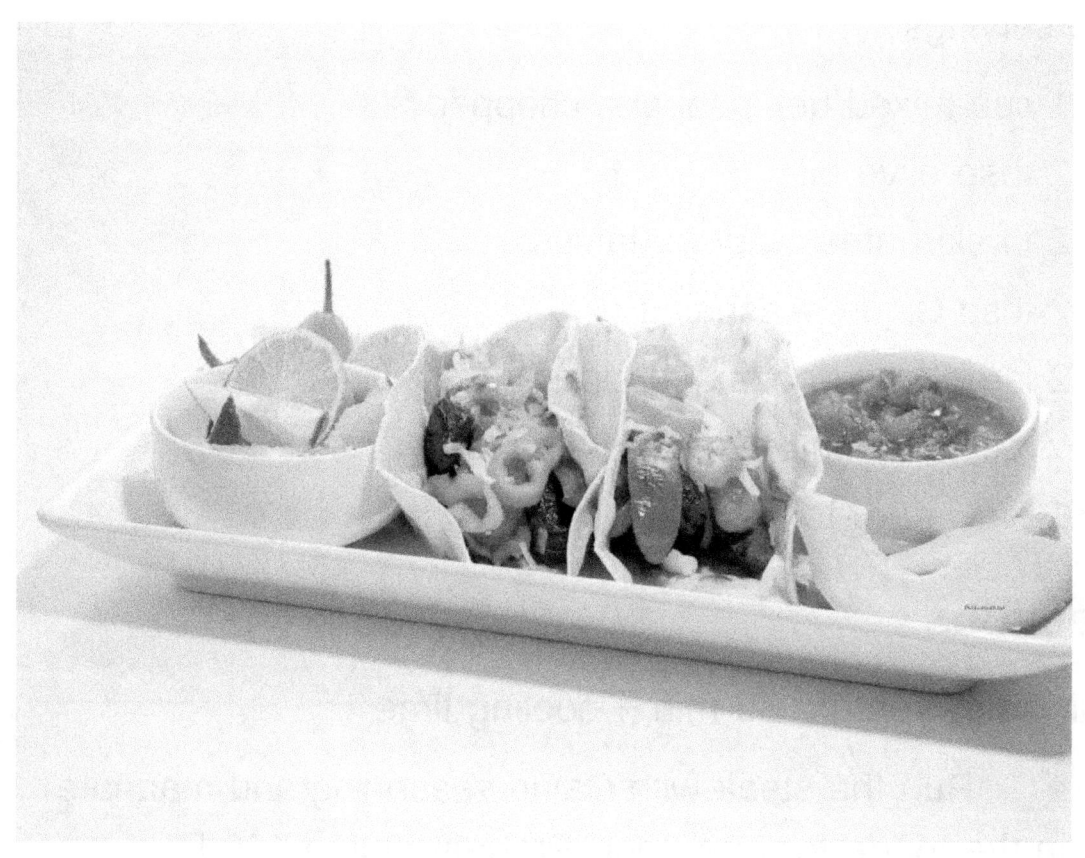

FISH & SEAFOOD

22. PARMESAN SHRIMP SCAMPI PIZZA

Ingredients

For 4 servings

- 3 tbsp olive oil
- 2 tbsp butter
- ½ lb shrimp, deveined
- ½ cup almond flour
- ¼ tsp salt
- 2 tbsp ground psyllium husk
- 2 garlic cloves, minced
- ¼ cup white wine
- ½ tsp dried basil
- ½ tsp dried parsley
- ½ lemon, juiced
- 2 cups grated cheese blend
- ½ tsp Italian seasoning
- ¼ cup grated Parmesan

Directions

Total Time: approx. 30 minutes

1. Preheat oven to 380 F. Line a baking sheet with parchment paper. In a bowl, mix almond flour, salt, psyllium powder, 1 tbsp of olive oil, and 1 cup of lukewarm water until dough forms.

2. Spread the mixture on the baking sheet and bake for 10 minutes.

3   Meanwhile, heat butter and the remaining olive oil in a skillet. Sauté garlic for 30 seconds. Mix in the wine and cook until it reduces by half. Stir in basil, parsley, and lemon juice. Stir in the shrimp and cook for 3 minutes.

4   Mix in the cheese blend and Italian seasoning. Let the cheese melt, 3 minutes. Spread the shrimp mixture on the crust and top with Parmesan cheese. Bake for 5 minutes or until the cheese melts. Slice and serve warm.

Per serving:

- Cal 419
- Net Carbs 3g
- Fats 29g
- Protein 23g

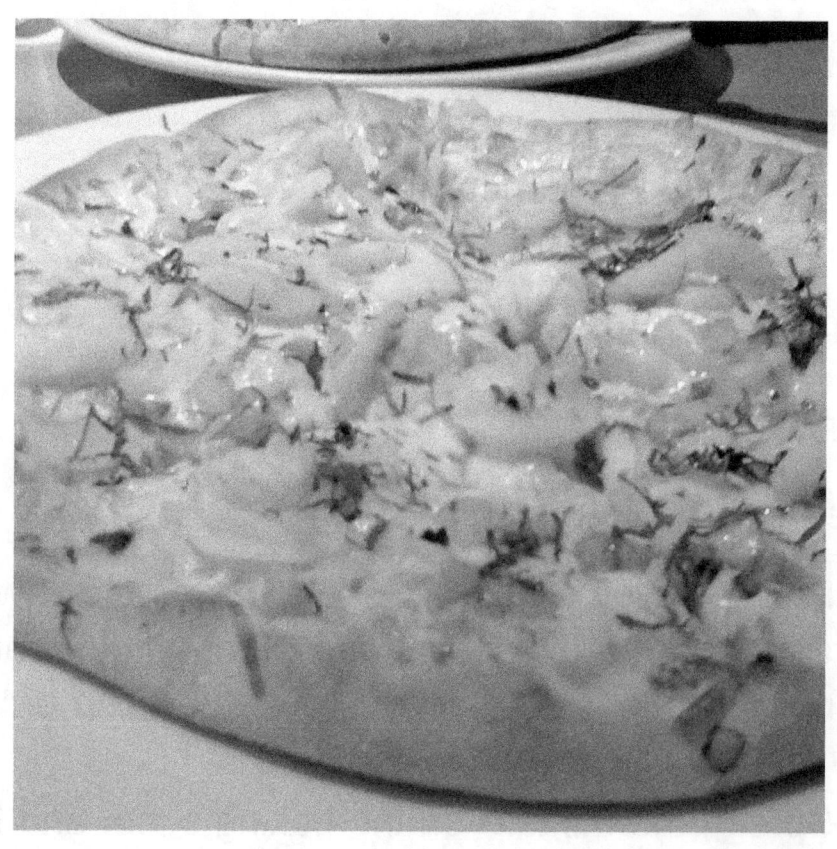

23. SPIRALIZED ZUCCHINI WITH GARLIC SHRIMP

Ingredients

For 4 servings

- 2 tbsp butter
- 1 lb jumbo shrimp, deveined
- 4 garlic cloves, minced
- 1 cup grated Parmesan cheese
- 1 pinch red chili flakes
- ¼ cup white wine
- 1 lime, zested and juiced
- 3 zucchinis, spiralized
- 2 tbsp chopped parsley
- Salt and black pepper to taste

Directions

Total Time: approx. 15 minutes

1. Warm the butter in a skillet and cook the shrimp for 3-4 minutes. Flip and stir in garlic and red chili flakes. Cook further for 1 minute; set aside.
2. Pour the wine and lime juice into the skillet and stir to deglaze the bottom; cook until reduced by a third.
3. Mix in zucchini, lime zest, shrimp, and parsley. Season with salt and pepper and cook for 2 minutes. Top with Parmesan and serve.

Per serving:

- Cal 261
- Net Carbs 8.9g
- Fats 8g
- Protein 29g

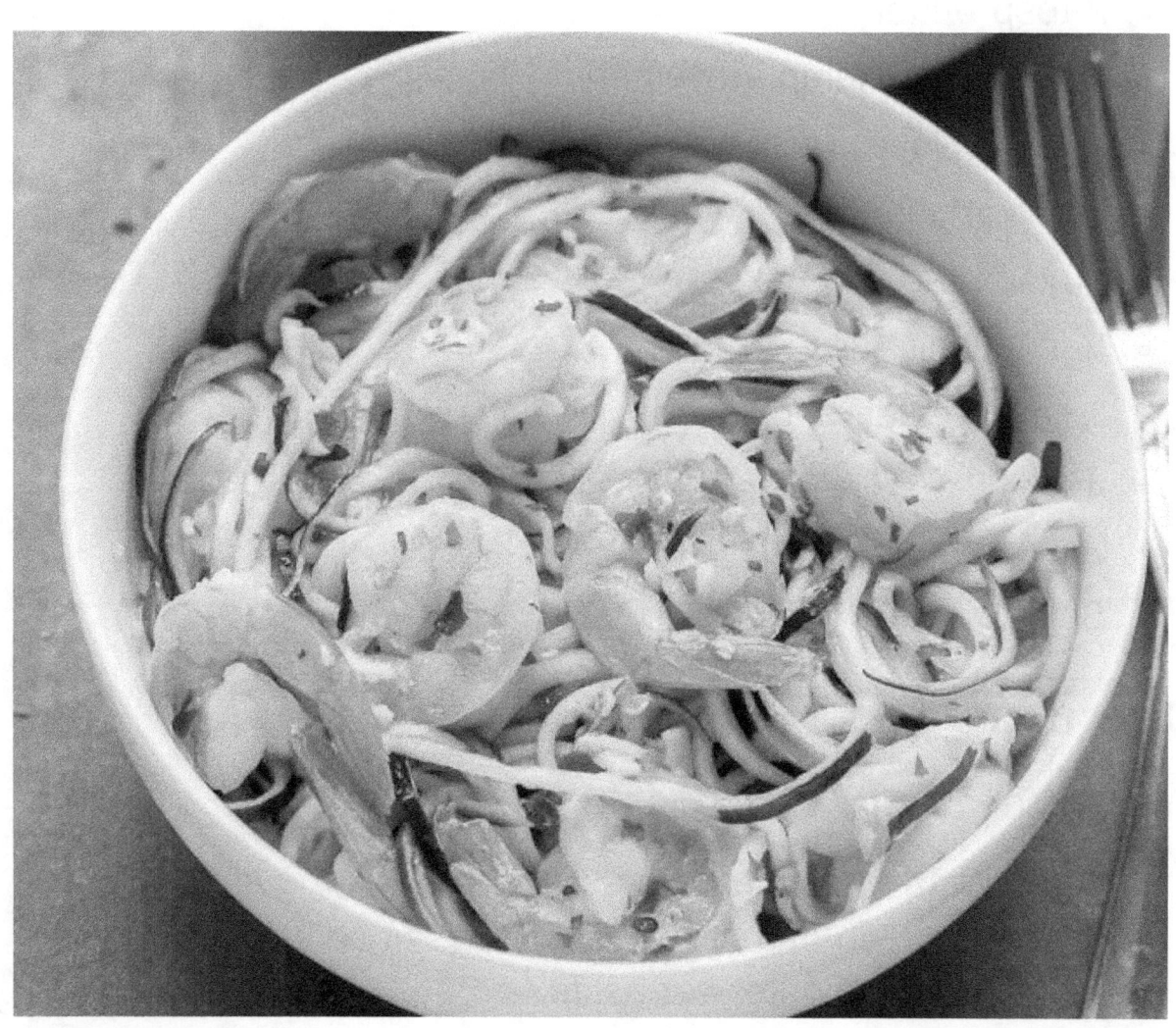

VEGETABLE SIDES & DAIRY

24. TOFU & PARSNIP SPAGHETTI A LA "BOLOGNESE"

Ingredients

For 4 servings

- 2 tbsp olive oil
- 2 tbsp butter
- 4 large parsnips, spiralized
- 1 cup crumbled firm tofu
- 1 onion, chopped
- 2 celery stalks, chopped
- 1 garlic clove, minced
- 2 cups sugar- free passata
- ¼ cup vegetable broth
- 2 tbsp fresh basil, chopped
- 1 cup grated Parmesan cheese
- Salt and black pepper to taste

Directions

Total Time: approx. 35 minutes

1   Warm butter in a skillet and sauté parsnips for 5 minutes. Season with salt and pepper: set aside.
2 Heat olive oil in a pot and cook tofu for 5 minutes.

3   Stir in onion, garlic, and celery and cook for 5 minutes. Mix in passata and broth and season with salt and pepper.

4   Cover the pot and cook until the sauce thickens, 8-10 minutes. Stir in basil. Divide the pasta between plates and

top with the sauce.

5   Sprinkle the Parmesan cheese on top and serve.

Per serving:

- Cal 431
- Net Carbs 31g
- Fats 19g
- Protein 22g

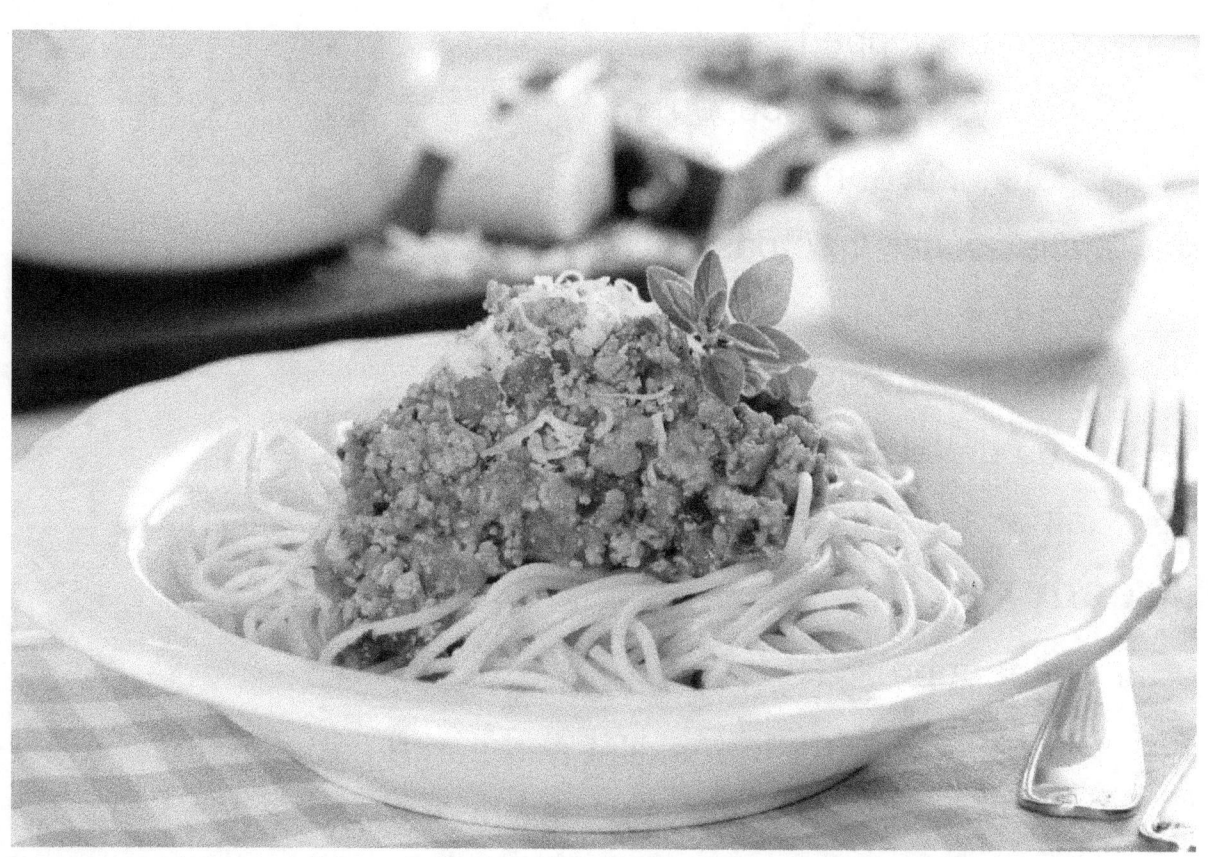

25. VEGETABLE KETO PASTA GRATIN

Ingredients

For 4 servings

- 1 cup shredded mozzarella cheese
- 1 cup sliced white button mushrooms
- 1 egg yolk
- 2 tbsp olive oil
- 1 cup chopped bell peppers
- 1 yellow squash, chopped
- 1 red onion, sliced
- Salt and black pepper to taste
- ¼ tsp red chili flakes
- 1 cup marinara sauce
- 1 cup grated mozzarella
- 1 cup grated Parmesan cheese

Directions

1. Total Time: approx. 35 min + chilling time

2. Place the mozzarella cheese in the microwave for 2 minutes. Take out the bowl and allow cooling for 1 minute. Mix in egg yolk until well-combined.

3. Lay a parchment paper on a flat surface, pour the cheese mixture on top, and cover with another parchment paper.

4. Flatten the dough into 1/8-inch thickness. Take off the parchment paper and cut the dough into penne-size pieces.

Place in a bowl and refrigerate overnight. Bring 2 cups of water to a boil and add in the "penne". Cook for 1 minute and drain; set aside.

5   Heat oil in a pan and sauté bell peppers, squash, onion, and mushrooms. Cook for 5 minutes. Season with salt, pepper, and chili flakes. Mix in marinara sauce and cook for 5 minutes. Stir in penne and spread the mozzarella and Parmesan cheeses on top. Bake for 15 minutes. Serve.

Per serving:

- Cal 250
- Net Carbs 5g
- Fats 12g
- Protein 31g

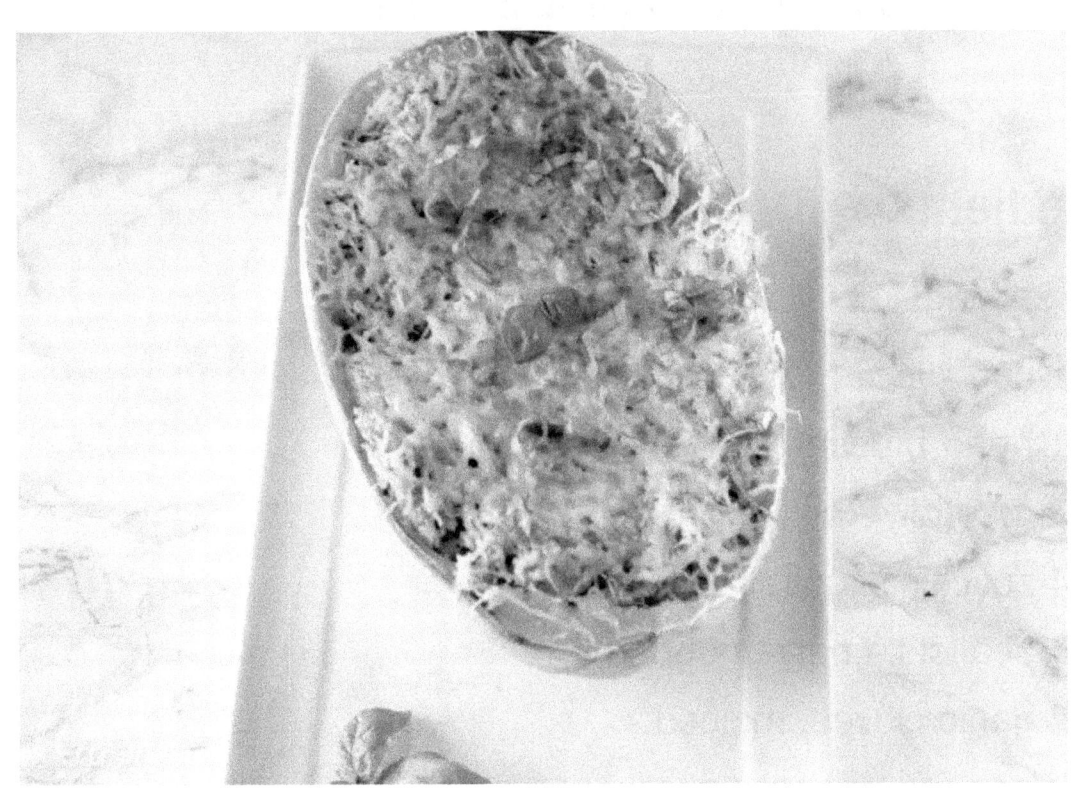

26. BALSAMIC ZOODLES WITH BROCCOLI & PEPPERS

Ingredients

For 4 servings

- 1 cup sliced mixed bell peppers
- 1 head broccoli, cut into florets
- 2 tbsp olive oil
- 4 zucchinis, spiralized
- 4 shallots, finely chopped
- 2 garlic cloves, minced
- ¼ tsp red pepper flakes
- 1 cup chopped kale
- 2 tbsp balsamic vinegar
- ½ lemon, juiced
- 1 cup grated Parmesan cheese
- Salt and black pepper to taste

Directions

Total Time: approx. 20 minutes

1   Warm oil in a skillet and sauté broccoli, bell peppers, and shallots until softened, 7 minutes.

2   Mix in garlic and red pepper flakes and cook until fragrant, 30 seconds. Stir in kale and zucchini spaghetti; cook until tender, 3 minutes. Mix in vinegar and lemon juice and adjust the taste with salt and pepper.

3   Garnish with Parmesan cheese. Serve.

Per serving:

- Cal 201
- Net Carbs 5.9g
- Fats 13g
- Protein 10g

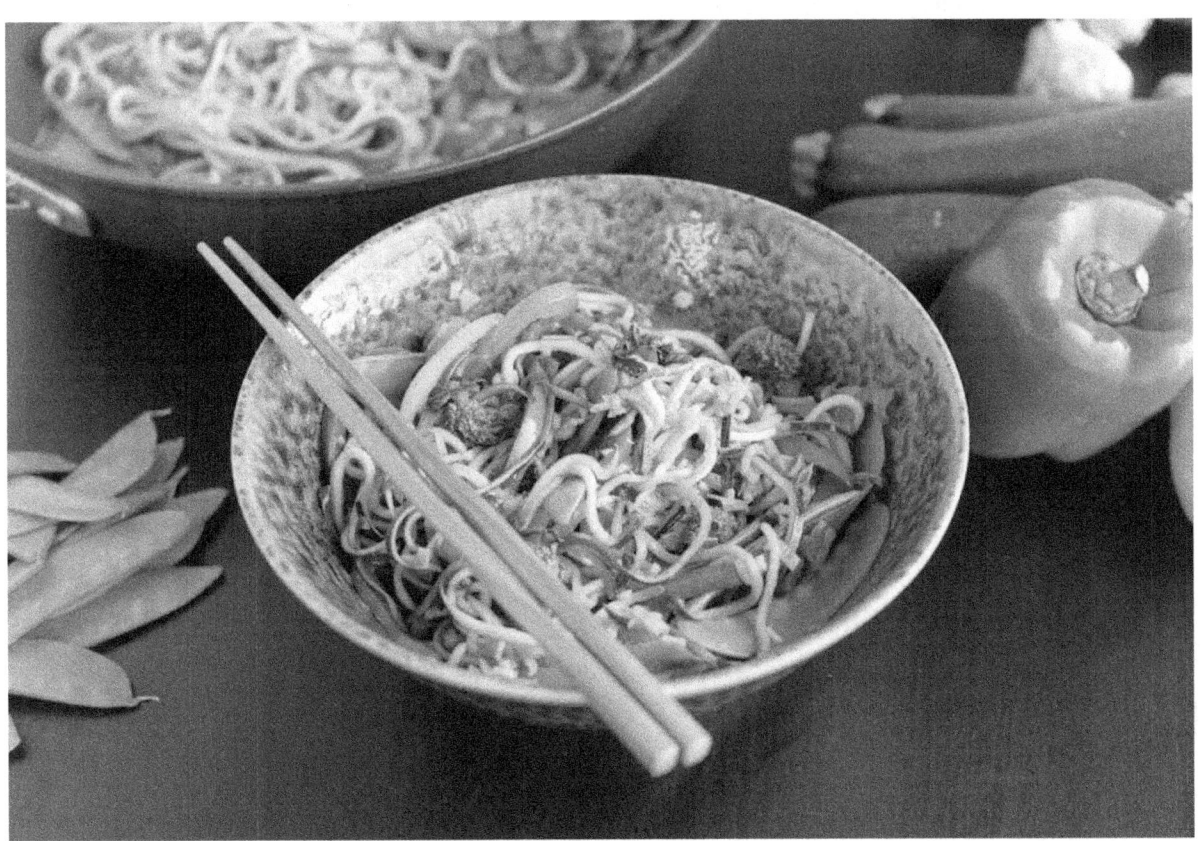

27. MUSHROOM & ZUCCHINI WITH SPINACH DIP

Ingredients

For 4 servings

Spinach Dip

- 3 oz spinach, chopped
- 1 avocado, halved and pitted
- 2 tbsp fresh lemon juice
- 1 garlic clove, minced
- 2 oz pecans
- Salt and black pepper to taste
- ¾ cup olive oil Zucchini
- 2 zucchinis, sliced
- Salt and black pepper to taste
- ½ lb mushrooms, sliced
- 2 tbsp olive oil

Directions

Total Time: approx. 20 minutes

1. Place the spinach in a food processor along with the avocado pulp, lemon juice, garlic, and pecans. Blend the ingredients until smooth, then season with salt and pepper. Add in olive oil and process a little more. Pour the pesto into a bowl; set aside. Place the zucchinis and mushrooms in a bowl. Season with salt, pepper, and oil.

2Preheat a grill pan over medium heat and cook both the mushroom and zucchini slices until browned on both sides. Plate the veggies and serve with spinach dip.

Per serving:

- Cal 683
- Fat 72g
- Net Carbs 5.5g
- Protein 5.3g

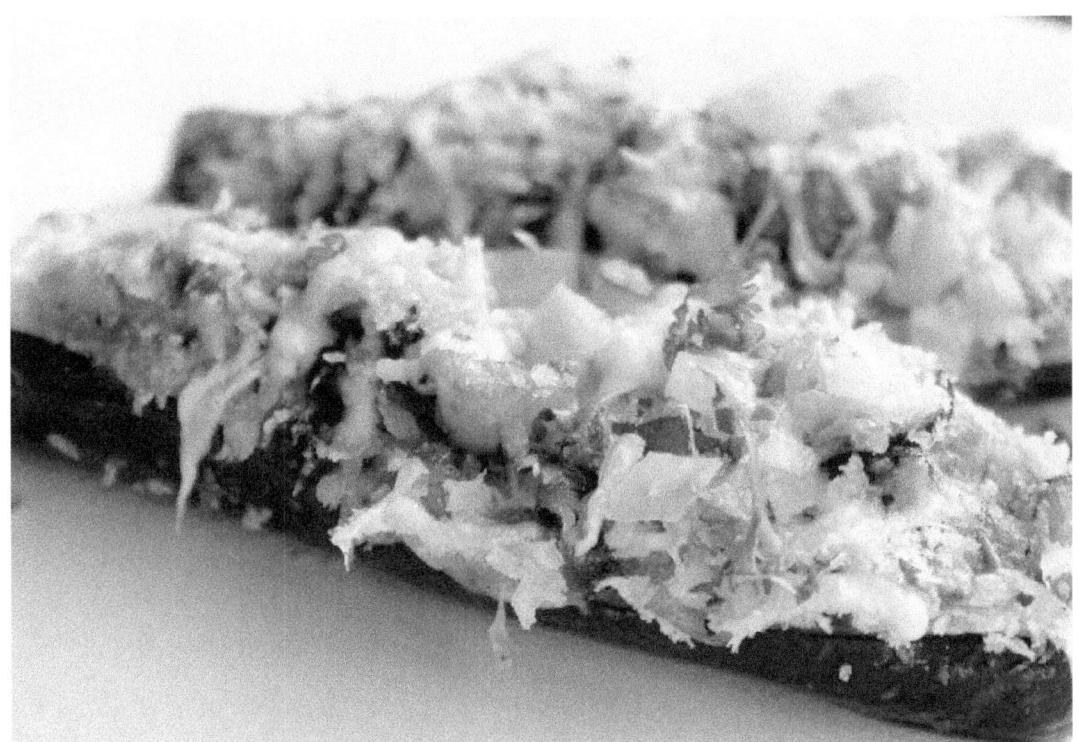

VEGAN

28. FENNEL & CELERIAC WITH CHILI TOMATO SAUCE

Ingredients

For 4 servings

- 2 tbsp olive oil
- 1 garlic clove, crushed
- ½ celeriac, sliced
- ½ fennel bulb, sliced
- ¼ cup vegetable stock
- Salt and black pepper to taste

Sauce

- 2 tomatoes, halved
- 2 tbsp olive oil
- ½ cup onions, chopped
- 2 cloves garlic, minced
- 1 chili, minced
- 1 bunch fresh basil, chopped
- 1 tbsp fresh cilantro, chopped
- Salt and black pepper to taste

Directions

Total Time: approx. 35 minutes

1. Set a pan over medium-high heat and warm olive oil. Sauté the garlic for 1 minute.

2   Stir in celeriac and fennel slices for 3-4 minutes, then pour in the stock; cook until softened, 5 minutes. Sprinkle with salt and pepper.

3   Brush the tomato halves with olive oil. Microwave for 15 minutes; get rid of any excess liquid.

4   Remove the cooked tomatoes to a food processor; add the ingredients for the sauce and puree to obtain the desired consistency.

5   Serve the celeriac and fennel topped with tomato sauce.

Per serving:

- Cal 145
- Fat 15g
- Net Carbs 5.3g
- Protein 2.1g

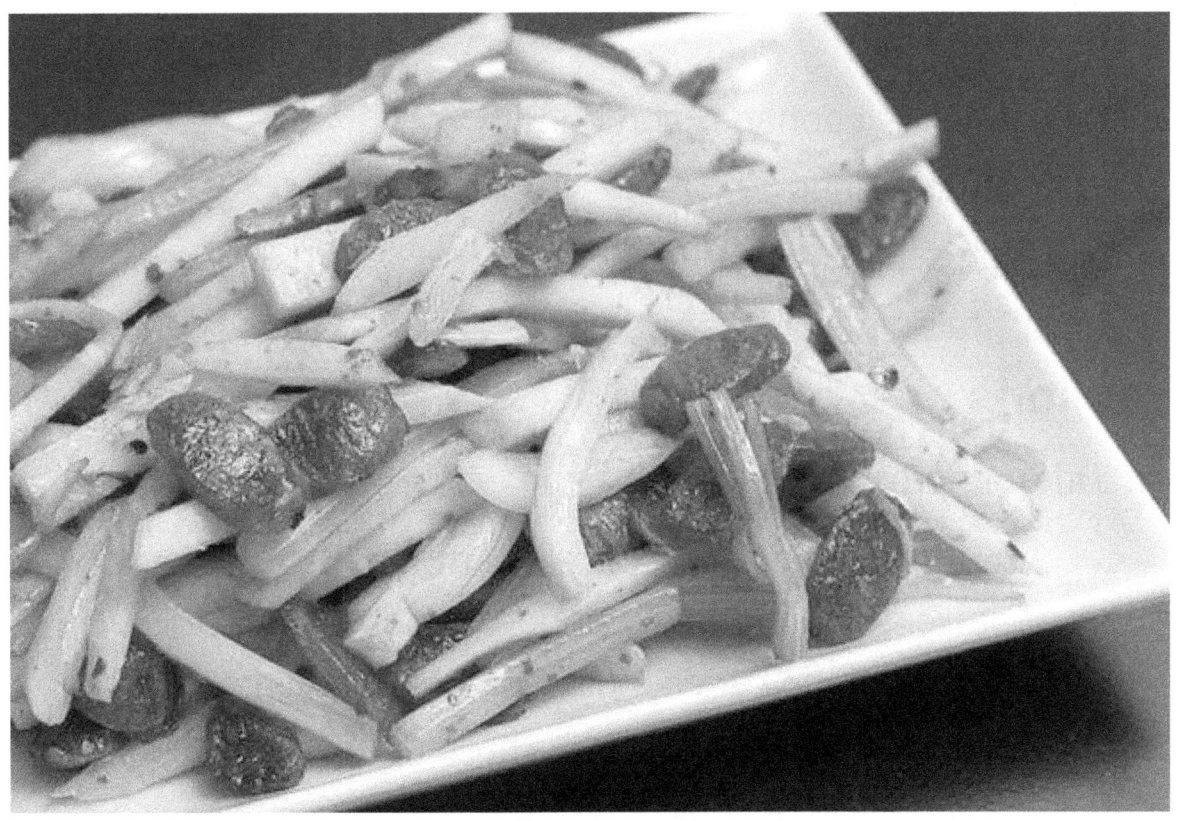

29. POPPY SEED COLESLAW

Ingredients

For 4 servings

Dressing

- 2 tbsp olive oil
- 1 cup poppy seeds
- 2 tbsp green onions, chopped
- 1 garlic clove, minced
- 1 lime, freshly squeezed
- Salt and black pepper to taste
- ¼ tsp dill, minced
- 1 tbsp yellow mustard

Salad

- ½ head white cabbage, shredded
- 1 carrot, shredded
- 1 shallot, sliced
- 2 tbsp Kalamata olives, pitted

Directions

Total Time: approx. 15 minutes

1   In a bowl, whisk the olive oil, mustard, lime juice, garlic, salt, and black pepper green onions.

2   Add the poppy seeds, dill, and green onions and mix well. Place cabbage, carrot, and shallot in a bowl and mix to

combine.

3   Transfer to a salad plate, pour the dressing over, and top with Kalamata olives to serve.

Per serving:

- Cal 235
- Fat 17g
- Net Carbs 6.4g
- Protein 8.1g

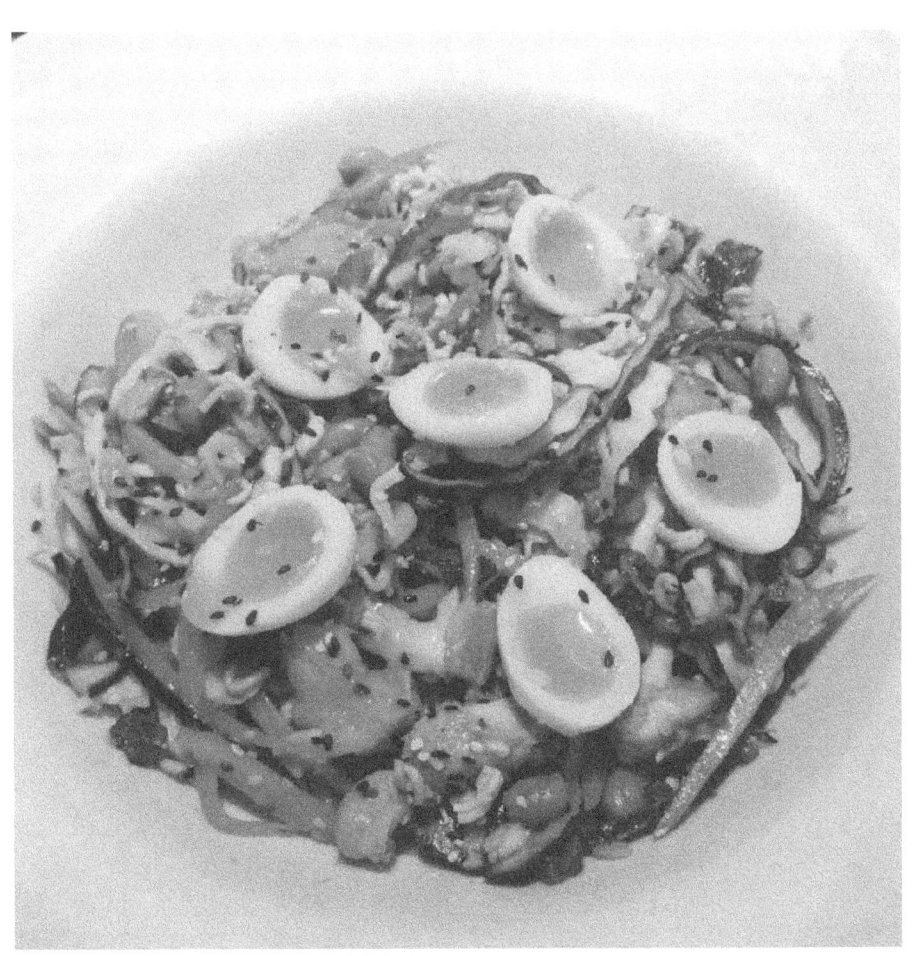

92

SNACKS & APPETIZERS

30. CHEESY BACON BITES

Ingredients

For 4 servings

- 6 oz cream cheese
- 6 oz shredded Gruyere cheese
- 7 bacon slices
- 2 tbsp butter, softened
- ½ tsp red chili flakes

Directions

Total Time: approx. 30 minutes

1   Place the bacon in a skillet and fry over medium heat until crispy, 5 minutes.

2   Transfer to a plate to cool and crumble it. Pour the bacon grease into a bowl and mix in cream cheese, Gruyere cheese, butter, and red chili flakes. Refrigerate to set for 15 minutes.

3   Remove and mold into walnutsized balls. Roll in the crumbled bacon. Plate and serve.

Per serving:

- Cal 541
- Net Carbs 0.5g
- Fat 49g
- Protein 22g

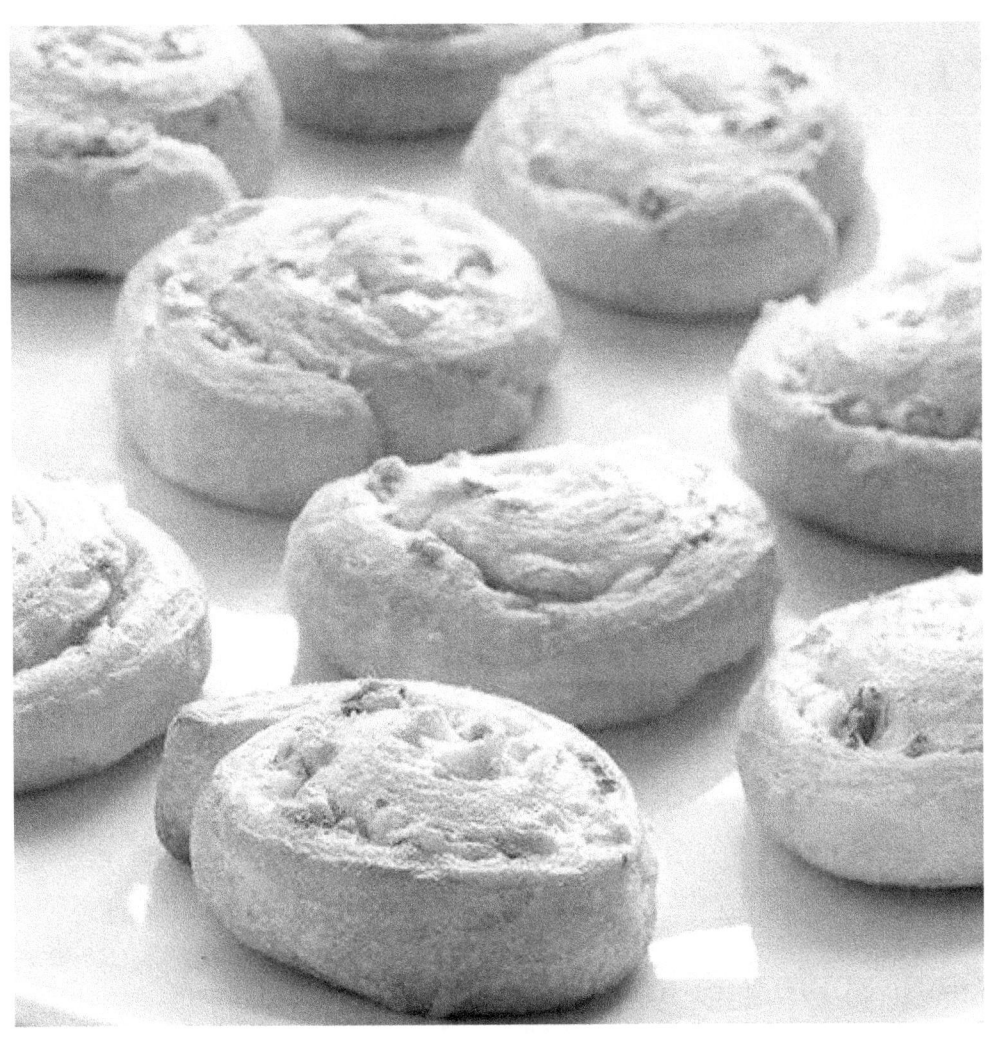

31. CHEESY GREEN BEAN & BACON ROAST

Ingredients

For 4 servings

- 1 egg, beaten
- 5 tbsp grated mozzarella
- 2 tbsp olive oil
- 1 tsp onion powder
- 15 oz fresh green beans
- 4 bacon slices, chopped

Directions

Total Time: approx. 30 minutes

1. Preheat oven to 360 F. Line a baking sheet with parchment paper. In a bowl, mix olive oil, onion powder, and egg.
2. Add in green beans and mozzarella and toss to coat.
3. Pour the mixture onto the baking sheet and bake until the cheese melts, 20 minutes.
4. Fry bacon in a skillet until crispy. Remove green beans and divide between serving plates. Top with bacon and serve.

Per serving:

- Cal 210
- Net Carbs 2.6g

- Fat 19g
- Protein 5.9g

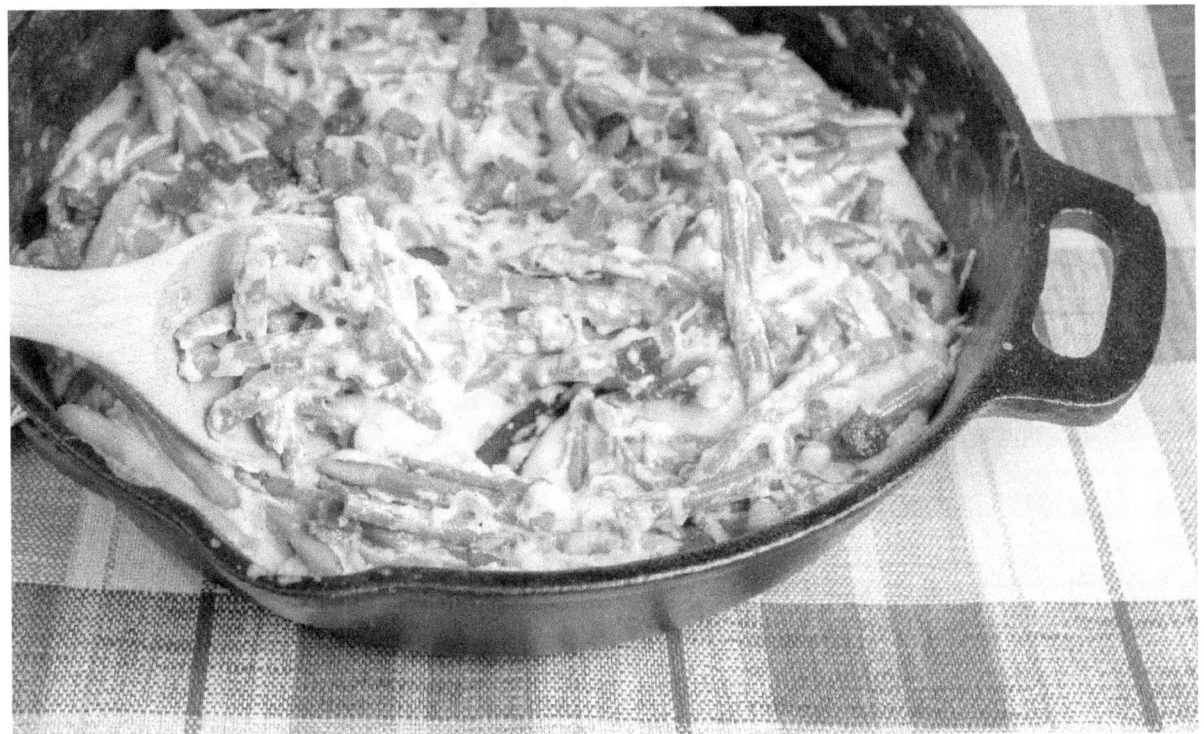

32. PARSLEY CAULIFLOWER & BACON STIR-FRY

Ingredients

For 4 servings

- 1 head cauliflower, cut into florets
- 10 oz bacon, chopped
- 1 garlic clove, minced
- 2 tbsp parsley, finely chopped
- Salt and black pepper to taste

Directions

Total Time: approx. 15 minutes

1   Throw the cauliflower in salted boiling water over medium heat and cook for 5 minutes or until soft; drain and set aside. In a skillet, fry bacon until brown and crispy, 5 minutes.

2   Add cauliflower and garlic and sauté until the cauliflower browns slightly.

3   Season with salt and pepper. Garnish with parsley and serve.

Per serving:

- Cal 239
- Net Carbs 3.9g
- Fat 21g
- Protein 8.9g

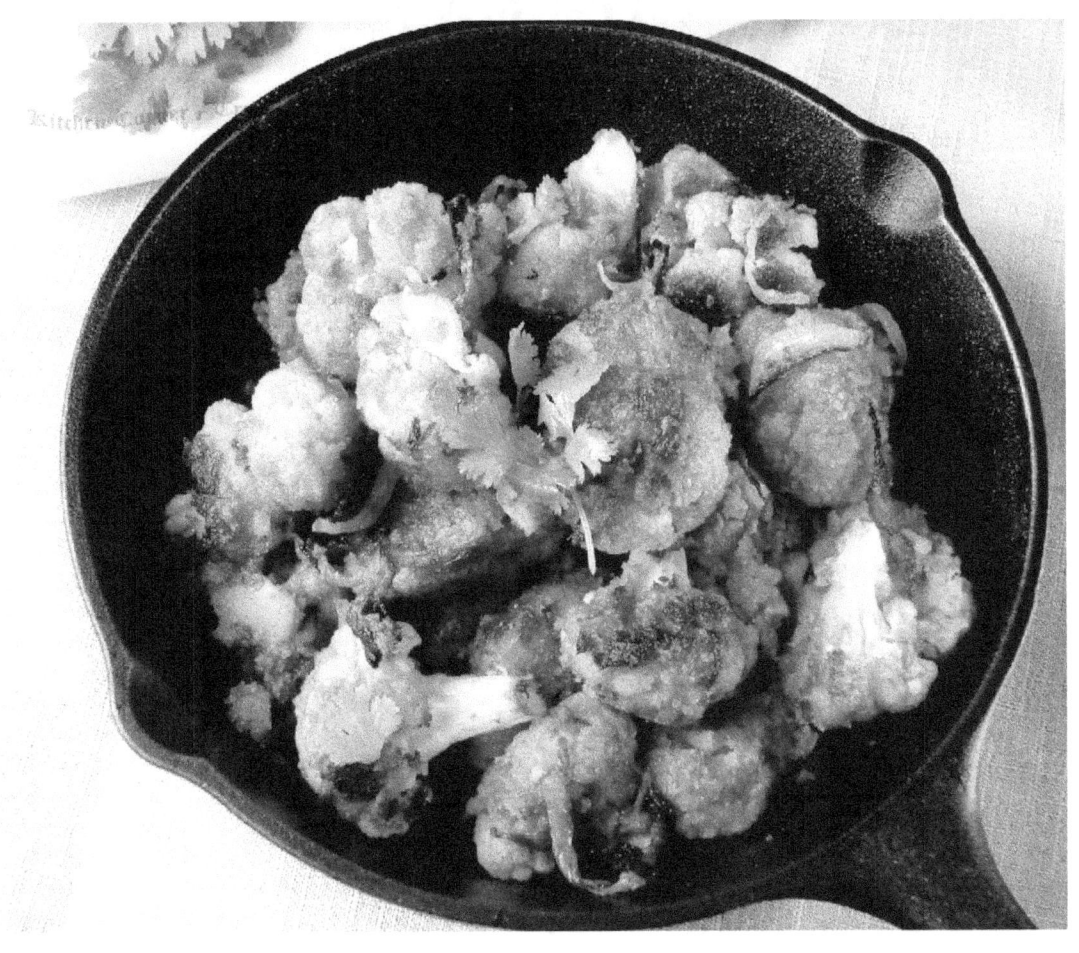

33. ARTICHOKE & BACON GRATIN WITH CAULI RICE

Ingredients

For 4 servings

- 1 cup canned artichoke hearts
- 6 bacon slices, chopped
- 2 cups cauliflower rice
- 3 cups baby spinach, chopped
- 1 garlic clove, minced
- 1 tbsp olive oil
- Salt and black pepper to taste
- ¼ cup sour cream
- 8 oz cream cheese, softened
- ¼ cup grated Parmesan
- 1 ½ cups grated mozzarella

Directions

Total Time: approx. 30 minutes

1   Drain and chop the artichokes; set aside. Preheat oven to 360 F. Cook bacon in a skillet over medium heat until brown and crispy, 5 minutes. Spoon onto a plate.

2   In a bowl, mix cauli rice, artichokes, spinach, garlic, olive oil, salt, pepper, sour cream, cream cheese, bacon, and half of Parmesan cheese.

3   Spread the mixture onto a baking dish and top with the remaining Parmesan and mozzarella cheeses.

4 Bake for 15 minutes.

5   Serve.

Per serving:

- Cal 498
- Net Carbs 5.3g
- Fat 41g
- Protein 28g

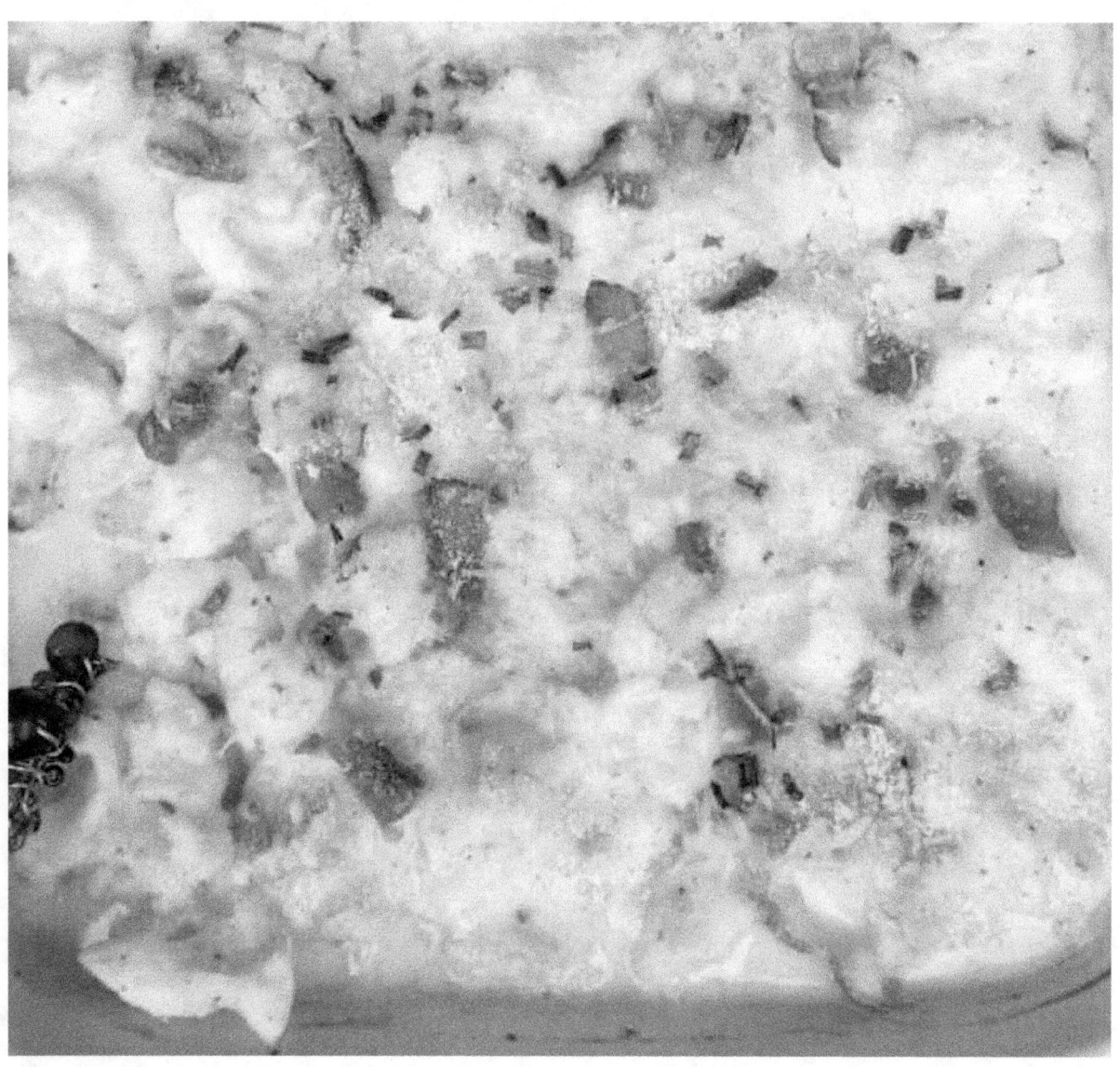

34. OREGANO PARSNIP MASH WITH HAM

Ingredients

For 4 servings

- 3 tbsp olive oil
- 4 tbsp butter
- 1 lb parsnips, diced
- 2 tsp garlic powder
- ¾ cup almond milk
- 4 tbsp heavy cream
- 6 slices deli ham, chopped
- 2 tsp freshly chopped oregano

Directions

Total Time: approx. 50 minutes

1   Preheat oven to 380 F. Spread parsnips on a baking sheet and drizzle with 2 tbsp olive oil.

2   Cover tightly with aluminum foil and bake until the parsnips are tender, 40 minutes.

3   Remove from the oven, take off the foil, and transfer to a bowl.

4   Add in garlic powder, almond milk, heavy cream, and butter. With an immersion blender, puree the ingredients until smooth. Fold in the ham and sprinkle with oregano. Serve.

Per serving:

- Cal 480
- Net Carbs 20g
- Fat 29g
- Protein 9.8g

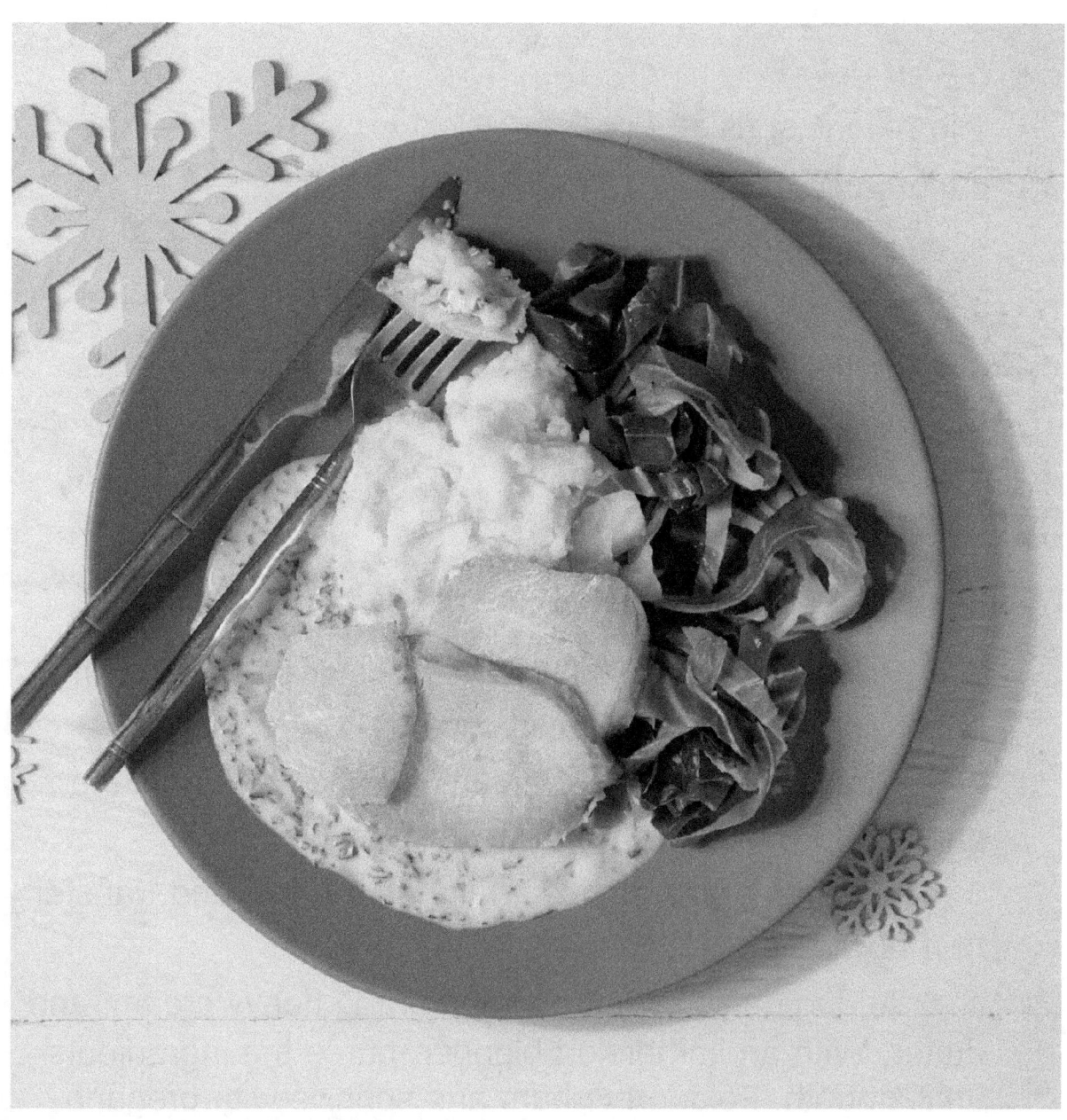

35. PANCETTA-WRAPPED STRAWBERRIES

Ingredients

For 4 servings

- 2 tbsp Swerve confectioner's sugar
- 12 fresh strawberries
- 12 thin pancetta slices
- 1 cup mascarpone cheese
- 1 /8 tsp white pepper

Directions

Total Time: approx. 30 minutes

1 In a bowl, combine mascarpone, Swerve confectioner's sugar, and white pepper.
2 Coat strawberries in the mixture, wrap each strawberry in a pancetta slice, and place on an ungreased baking sheet.
3 Bake in the oven at 425 F for 15-20 minutes until pancetta browns. Serve warm.

Per serving:

- Cal 169
- Net Carbs 1.2g
- Fat 11 g
- Protein 12g

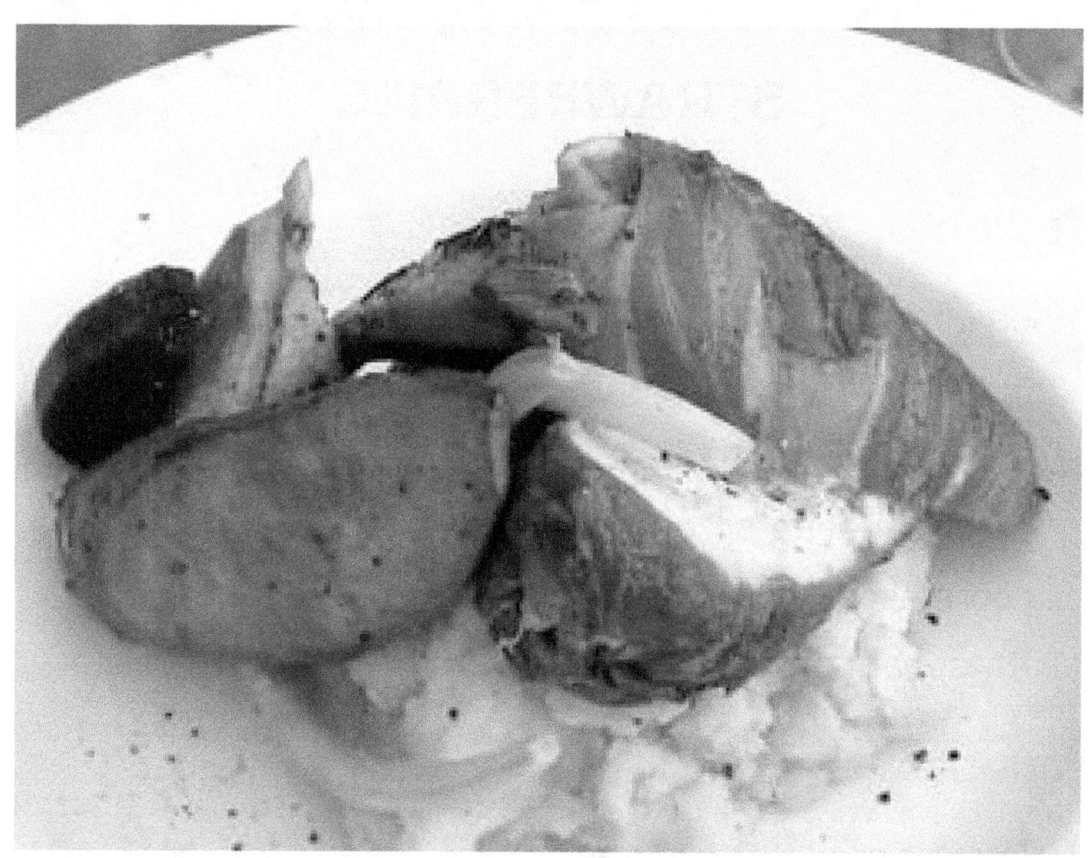

36. SPICY CAULIFLOWER FALAFEL

Ingredients

For 2 servings

- 1 head cauliflower, cut into florets
- 1 /3 cup silvered ground almonds
- 4 tbsp olive oil
- ½ tsp ground cumin
- 1 tsp parsley, chopped
- Salt to taste
- 1 tsp chili pepper
- 3 tbsp coconut flour
- 2 eggs

Directions

Total Time: approx. 20 minutes

1   Blitz the cauliflower in a food processor until a grain meal consistency is formed.

2   Transfer to a bowl, add in the ground almonds, ground cumin, parsley, salt, chili pepper, and coconut flour, and mix until evenly combined.

3   Beat the eggs in a bowl and mix with the cauli mixture. Shape ¼ cup each into patties and set aside.

4   Warm olive oil in a frying pan over medium heat and fry the patties for 5 minutes on each side until firm and browned.

5   Remove onto a wire rack to cool, share into serving plates, and serve.

Per serving:

- Cal 343
- Fat 31g
- Net Carbs 3.7g
- Protein 8.5g

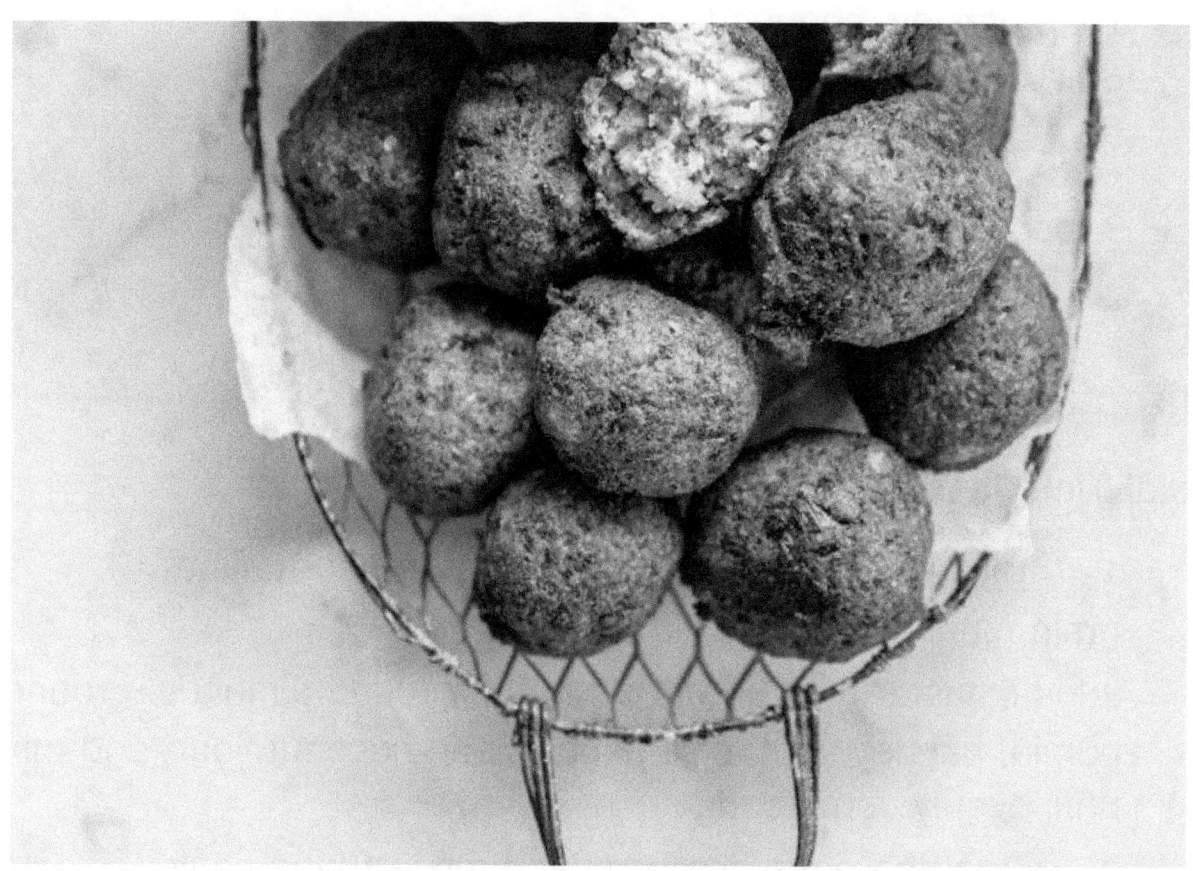

SMOOTHIES & BEVERAGES

37. ALMOND-RASPBERRY SMOOTHIE

Ingredients

For 4 servings

- ½ cup raspberries
- 1 ½ cups almond milk
- ½ tsp almond extract
- Juice from half lemon

Directions

Total Time: approx. 5 minutes

1. In a smoothie maker or blender, pour the almond milk, raspberries, lemon juice, and almond extract.
2. Puree the ingredients at high speed until the raspberries have blended almost entirely into the liquid.
3. Serve.

Per serving:

- Cal 408
- Net Carbs 9g
- Fat 39g
- Protein 5g

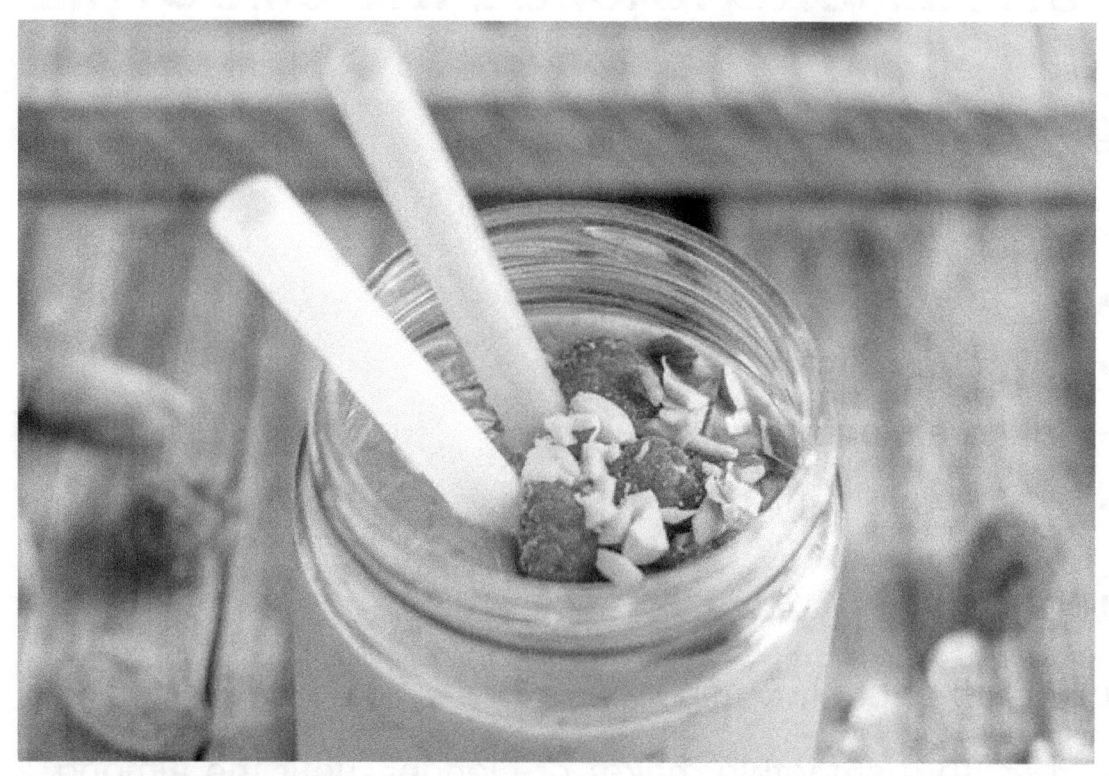

SWEETS & DESSERTS

38. CHOCOLATE AVOCADO TRUFFLES

Ingredients

For 6 servings

- 5 oz dark chocolate
- 1 tbsp coconut oil
- 1 ripe avocado, pitted
- 1 tbsp cocoa powder
- ½ tsp vanilla extract
- ½ tsp lemon zest

Directions

Total Time: approx. 15 minutes

1. Place the flesh of the avocado into a bowl and mix with vanilla using an immersion blender.
2. Stir in lemon zest. Microwave chocolate and coconut oil for 1 minute. Add to the avocado mixture and stir.
3. Allow cooling to firm up a bit. Form balls out of the mix. Roll each ball in the cocoa powder and serve immediately.

Per serving:

- Cal 69
- Net Carbs 2g
- Fat 5.9g
- Protein 1.8g

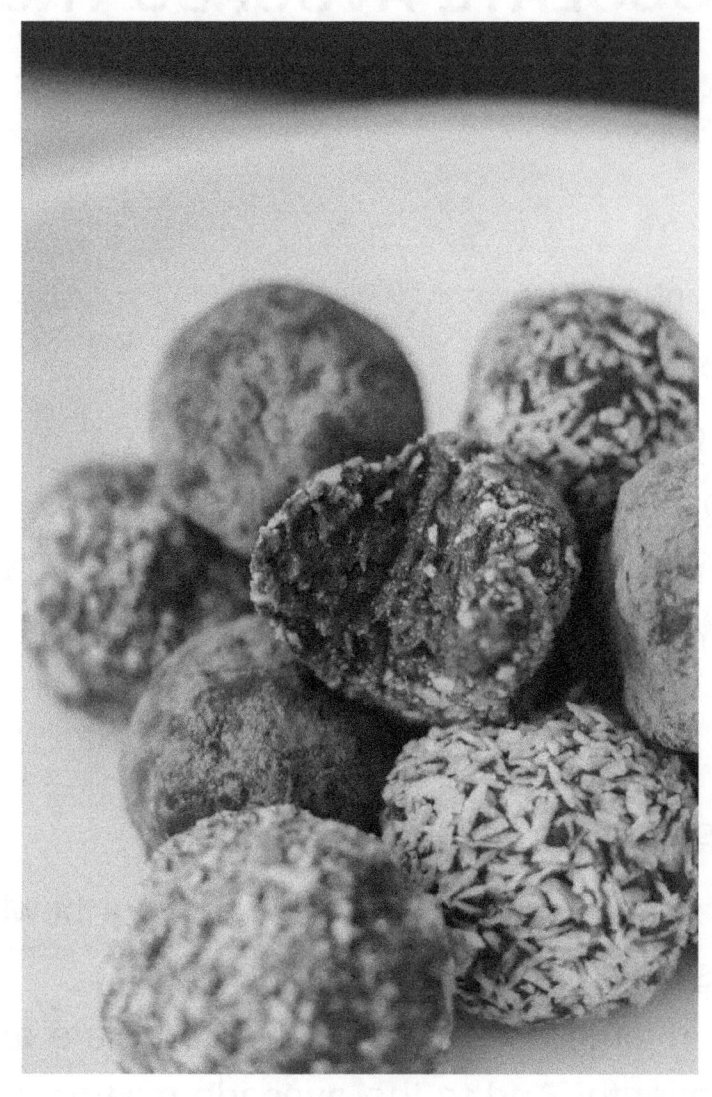

39. COCONUT FAT BOMBS

Ingredients

For 6 servings

- ½ cup grated coconut
- 3 oz butter, softened
- ¼ tsp cardamom powder
- ½ tsp vanilla extract
- ¼ tsp cinnamon powder

Directions

Total Time: approx. 15 min + chilling time

1. Place grated coconut into a skillet over medium heat and roast until lightly brown, about 1 minute; set aside.
2. In a bowl, combine butter, half of the coconut, cardamom, vanilla, and cinnamon.
3. Form balls from the mixture and roll each in the remaining coconut. Serve cooled.

Per serving:

- Cal 91
- Net Carbs 1g
- Fat 10g
- Protein 1g

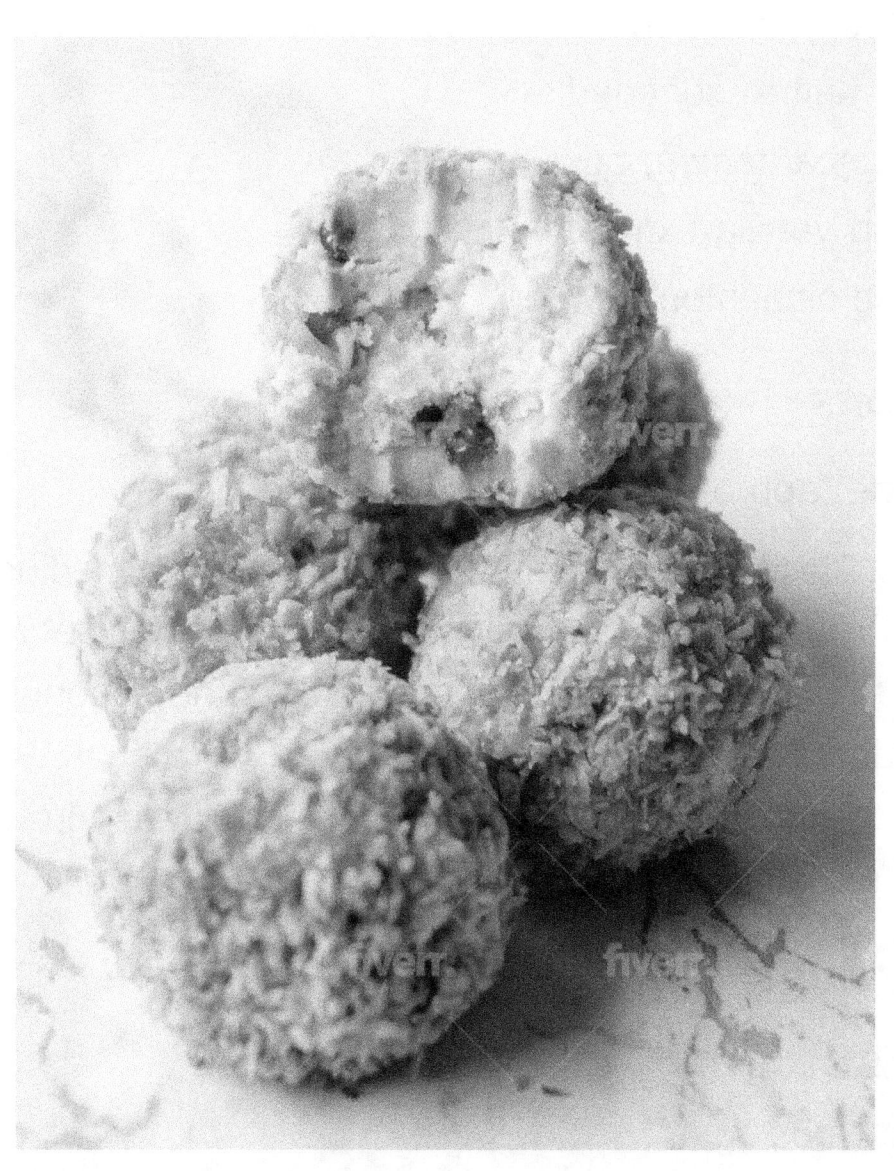

40. MAPLE-BERRY FAT BOMBS

Ingredients

For 4 servings

- 1 cup cranberries
- 1 cup strawberries
- 1 cup raspberries
- 2 tbsp sugar- free maple syrup
- 1 tsp vanilla extract
- 16 oz cream cheese, softened
- 4 tbsp unsalted butter

Directions

Total Time: approx. 20 min + chilling time

1. Puree the fruits in a blender with the vanilla. In a saucepan, melt cream cheese and butter together over medium heat and stir until mixed.
2. In a bowl, combine the berries, cheese mixtures, and maple syrup evenly. Line a muffin tray with liners.
3. Fill the muffin tray with the mix. Refrigerate for 40 minutes and serve.

Per serving:

- Cal 231
- Net Carbs 3.1g
- Fat 15g
- Protein 3.9g

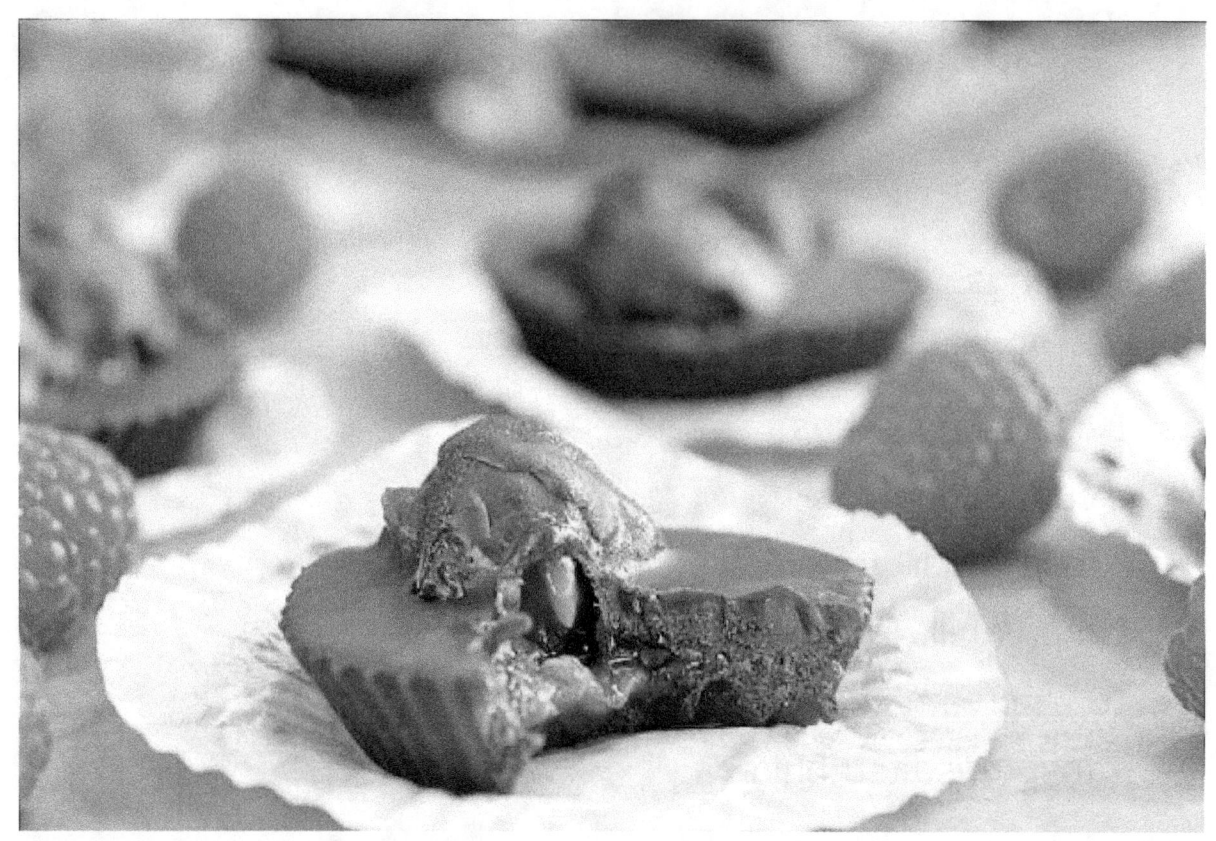

41. PEANUT BUTTER FAT BOMBS

Ingredients

For 4 servings

- ½ cup coconut oil
- ½ cup peanut butter
- 4 tbsp cocoa powder
- ½ cup erythritol

Directions

Total Time: approx. 10 min + cooling time

1. Warm butter and coconut oil in the microwave for 45 seconds, stirring twice until properly melted.
2. Mix in cocoa powder and erythritol until completely combined. Pour into muffin molds and refrigerate for 3 hours to harden.
3. Serve and enjoy!

Per serving:

- Cal 189
- Net Carbs 2g
- Fat 18g
- Protein 3.9g

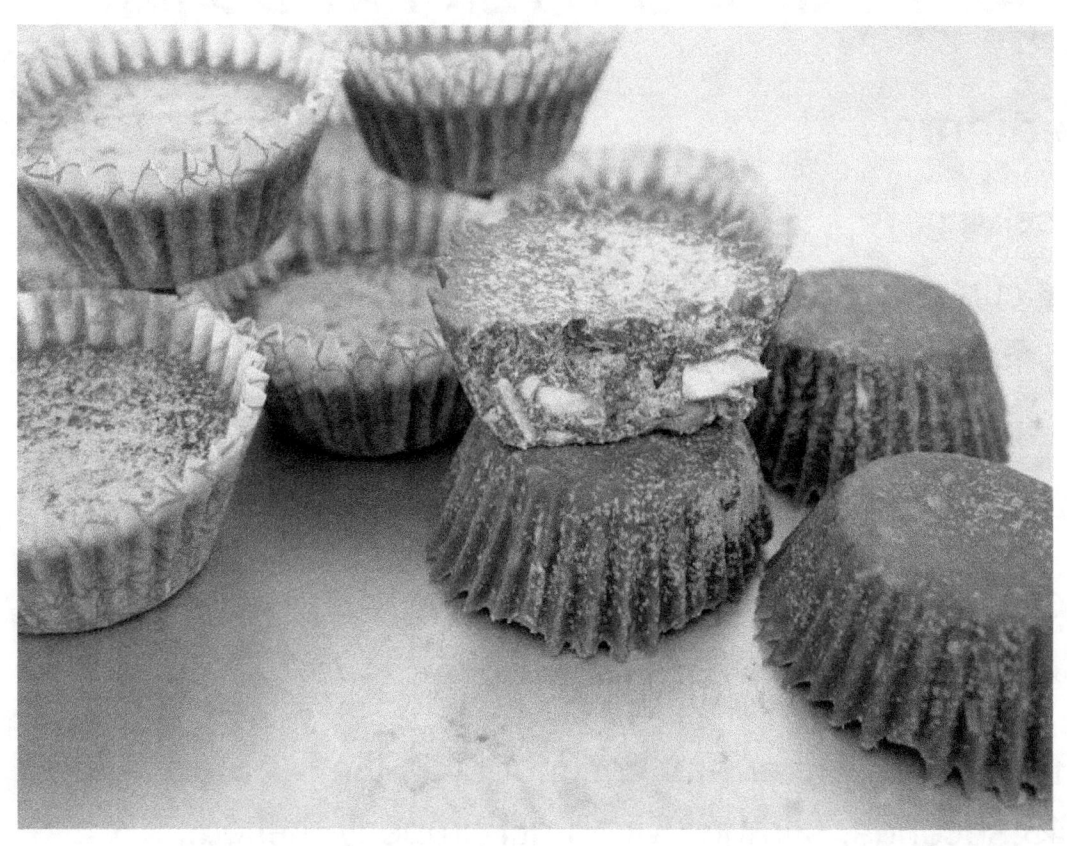

42. CHEESY FAT BOMBS WITH BREWED COFFEE

Ingredients

For 4 servings

- 1 cup cottage cheese
- ¼ cup melted butter
- 1 tbsp cocoa powder
- 2 tbsp xylitol
- 3 tbsp brewed coffee

Directions

Total Time: approx. 10 min + cooling time

1. In a bowl, whisk the cottage cheese, butter, cocoa powder, xylitol, and coffee with a hand mixer until creamy and fluffy, for about a minute.
2. Fill into muffin tins and freeze for 4 hours until firm.

Per serving:

- Cal 153
- Fat 14g
- Net Carbs 3.2g
- Protein 4.5g

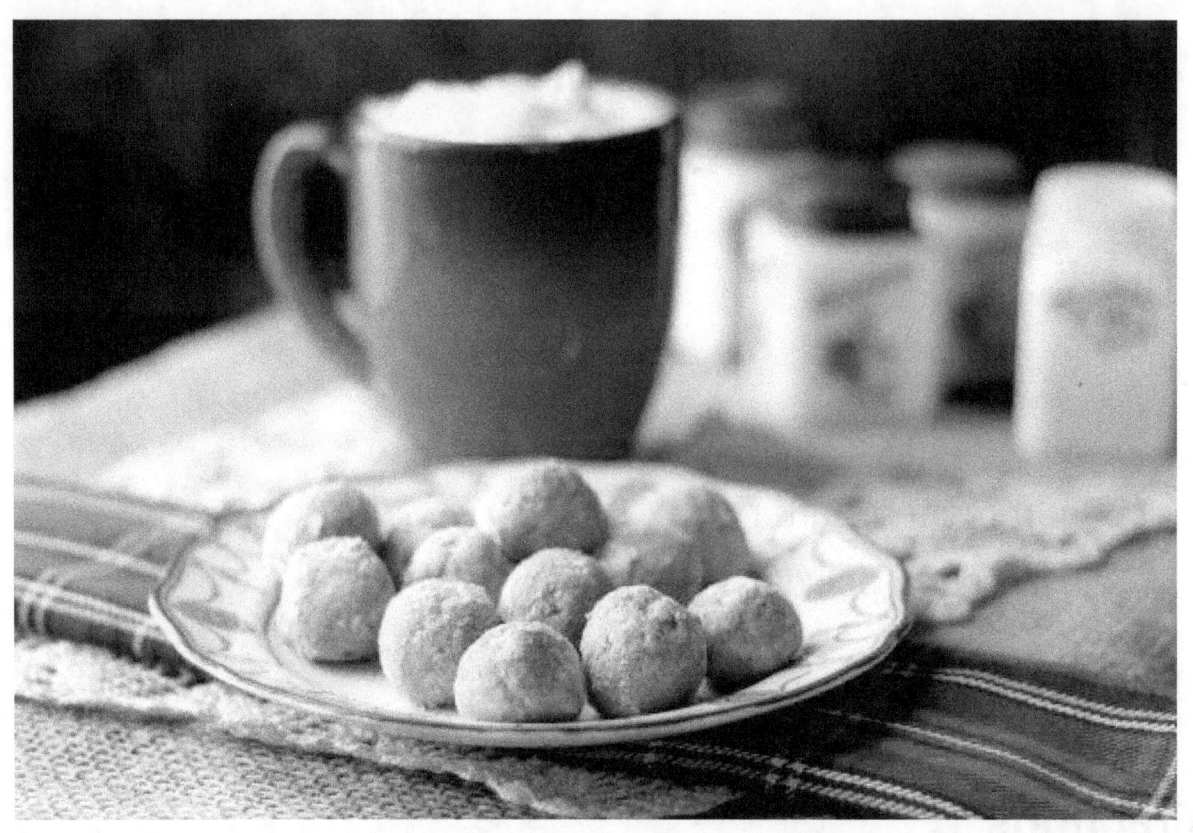

43. STRAWBERRY TRIFLE WITH HAZELNUTS

Ingredients

For 4 servings

- 3 oz fresh strawberries
- 2 oz toasted hazelnuts
- 1 ½ ripe avocados
- ¾ cup coconut cream
- Zest and juice of ½ a lemon
- 1 tbsp vanilla extract

Directions

Total Time: approx. 10 minutes

1. In a bowl, add avocado pulp, coconut cream, lemon zest and juice, and half of the vanilla extract.
2. Mix with an immersion blender. Put the strawberries and remaining vanilla in another bowl and use a fork to mash the fruit.
3. In a tall glass, alternate layering the cream and strawberry mixtures. Drop a few hazelnuts on each and serve.

Per serving:

- Cal 359
- Net Carbs 7g
- Fat 33.9g

- Protein 3.8g

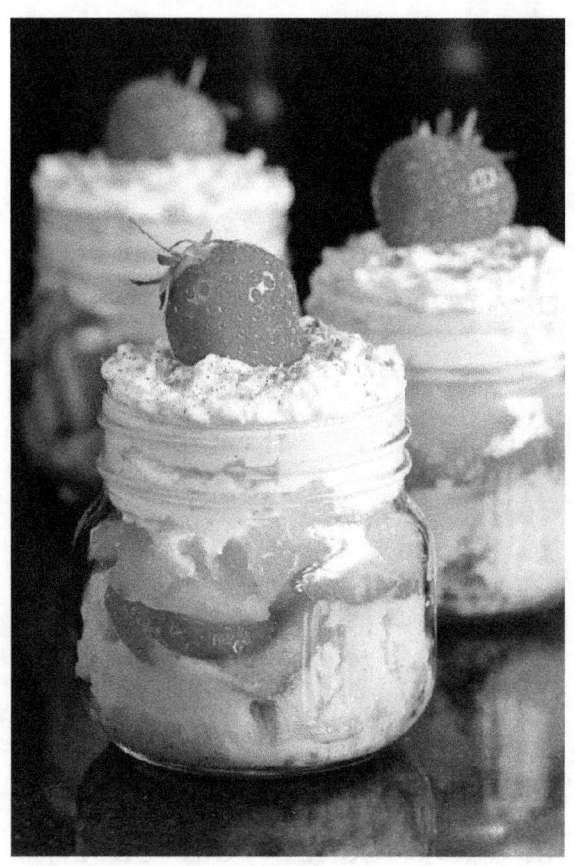

44. NO-BAKE PEANUT BUTTER COOKIES

Ingredients

For 4 servings

- ¾ cup peanut butter
- ¾ cup coconut oil
- 2 tbsp hulled hemp seeds
- ¼ cup cocoa powder
- 1 cup Swerve brown sugar
- 1 tsp vanilla extract
- 1 ½ cup coconut flakes

Directions

Total Time: approx. 25 minutes

1. Preheat oven to 360 F. Line two baking sheets with parchment paper. Add coconut oil and peanut butter to a pot.
2. Melt the mixture over low heat until smoothly combined.
3. Stir in cocoa powder, Swerve sugar, and vanilla until smooth.
4. Slightly increase the heat and simmer the mixture with occasional stirring until slowly boiling. Turn the heat off. Mix in coconut flakes and hemp seeds.
5. Set the mixture aside to cool. Spoon the batter into silicone muffin cups and freeze for 15 minutes or until set. Serve.

Per serving:

- Cal 359
- Net Carbs 5.5g
- Fat 37g
- Protein 4.7g

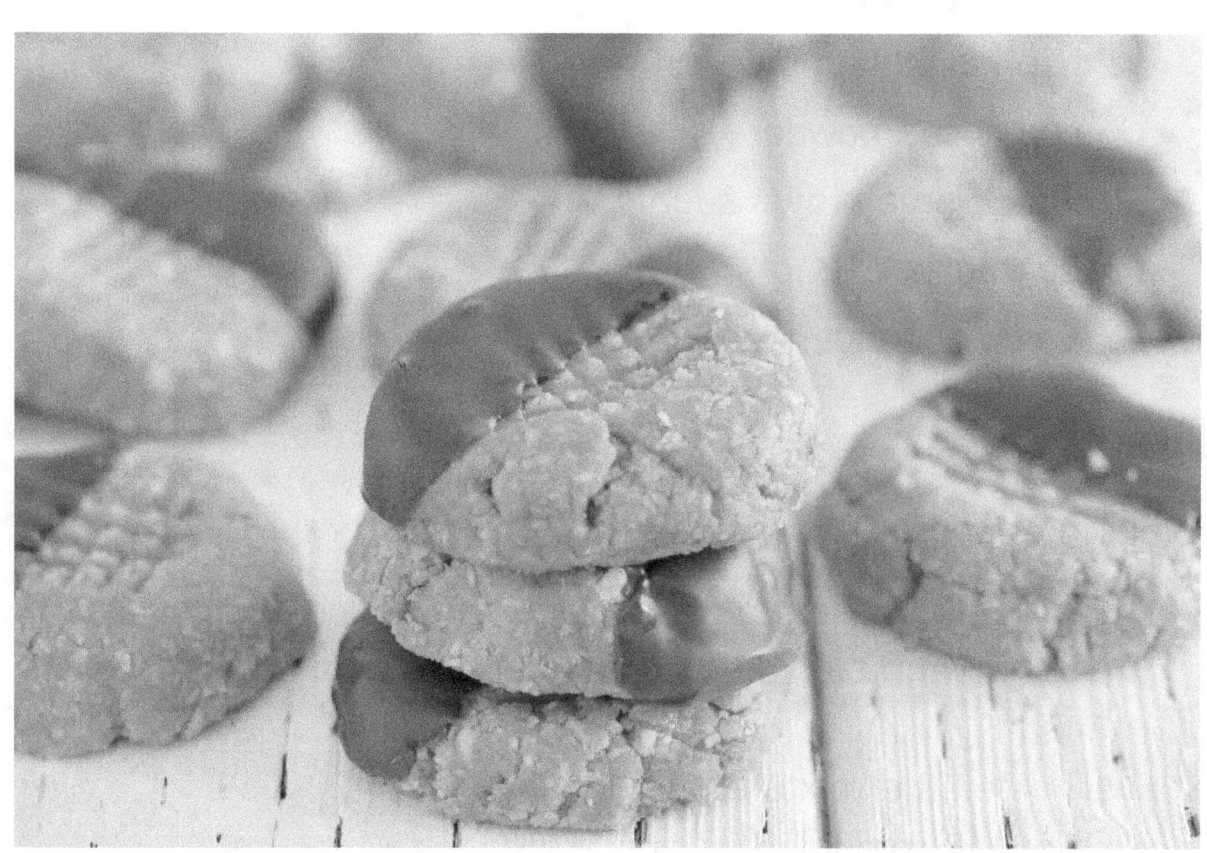

45. CHORIZO & CABBAGE BAKE

Ingredients

For 4 servings

- 1 head green cabbage, cut into wedges
- 1 lb chorizo, sliced
- 4 tbsp butter, melted
- Salt and black pepper to taste
- 2 tbsp Parmesan cheese, grated
- 1 tbsp parsley, chopped

Directions

Total Time: approx. 25 minutes

1. Preheat oven to 390 F and grease a baking tray with cooking spray.
2. Mix the butter, salt, and black pepper until evenly combined in a bowl.
3. Brush the mixture on all sides of the cabbage wedges.
4. Place on the baking sheet, add in the chorizo, and bake for 20 minutes to soften the cabbage.
5. Sprinkle with Parmesan cheese and parsley.

Per serving:

- Cal 268
- Fat 19g
- Net Carbs 4g

- Protein 17.5g

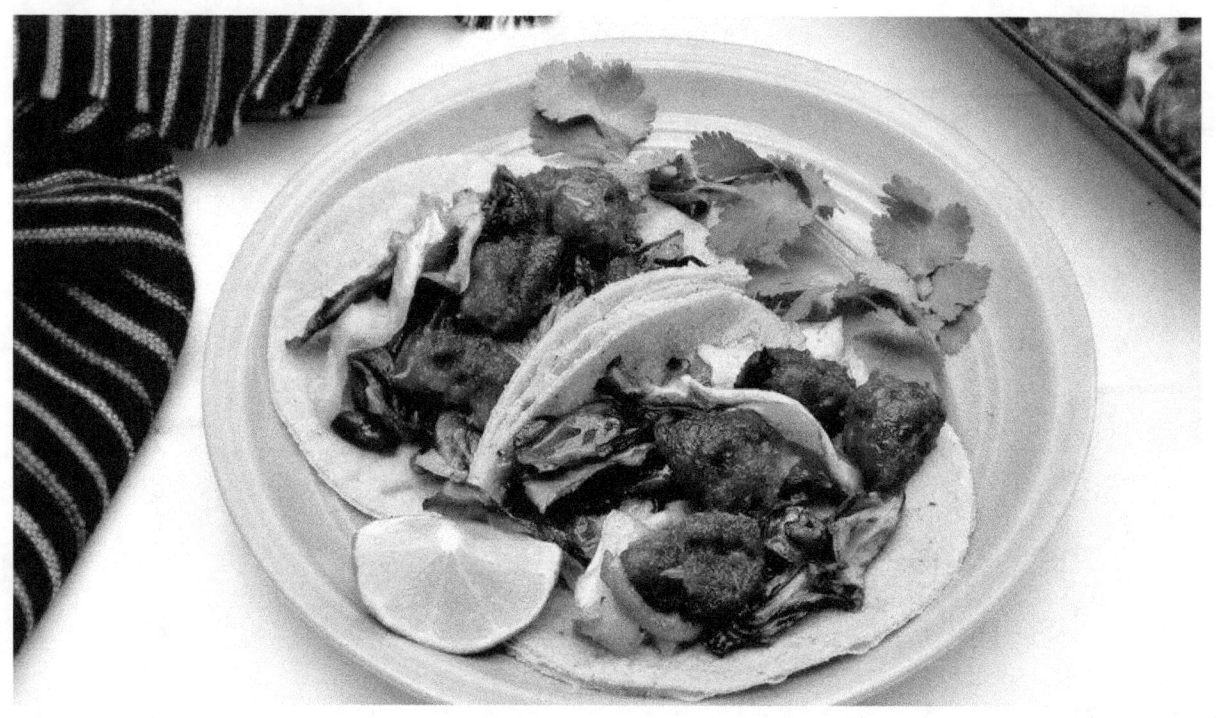

KETO SMALL APPLIANCE RECIPES

46. SLOW COOKER TURNIP SOUP WITH SOUR CREAM

Ingredients

For 4 servings

- 2 tbsp olive oil
- 1 cup onion, chopped
- 1 celery, chopped
- 2 garlic cloves, minced
- 2 turnips, peeled and chopped
- 3 cups vegetable broth
- ¼ cup ground almonds
- 1 cup almond milk
- 1 tbsp fresh cilantro, chopped
- 4 tsp sour cream

Directions

Total Time: approx. 8 hours 30 minutes

1 Warm the olive oil in a skillet over medium heat and sauté celery, garlic, and onion for 6 minutes.

2 Transfer to your slow cooker. Pour in the broth and turnips. Close the cover and cook on Low for 8 hours.

3 When ready, puree the soup with an immersion blender. Stir in the ground almonds and almond milk.

4   Serve garnished with sour cream and cilantro.

Per serving:

- Cal 125
- Fat 7.1g
- Net Carbs 7.7g
- Protein 4g

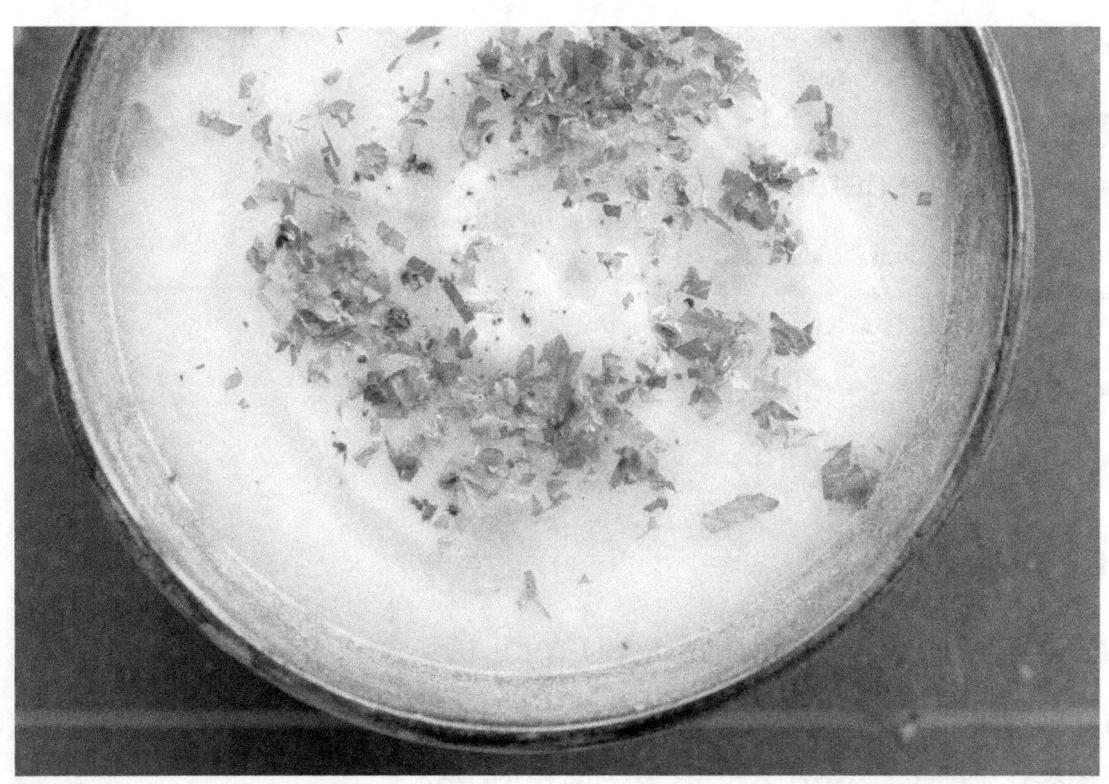

47. INSTANT POT CHICKEN LAZONE

Ingredients

For 6 servings

- 3 tsp garlic powder
- 2 tsp onion powder
- 2 tsp paprika
- 2 tsp Cayenne powder
- Salt and black pepper to taste
- 2 lb chicken strips
- 3 tbsp butter
- 3 tbsp olive oil
- 1 ⅓ cups chicken broth
- 2 cups heavy cream
- 3 tbsp chopped parsley

Directions

Total Time: approx. 45 minutes

1. Add the onion powder, salt, pepper, cayenne pepper, garlic powder, and paprika to a large bowl, and mix.
2. Rub the spices onto the chicken. Select Sauté on your Instant Pot. Warm the oil and butter and add the chicken pieces; brown them for about 10 minutes.
3. Pour in the chicken broth. Close the lid, secure the pressure valve, and select Manual on High Pressure. Cook for 15

minutes.

4. Once the timer has stopped, quickly release the pressure and open the lid. Select Saute and add the heavy cream.
5. Stir and cook until the sauce slightly thickens. Dish sauce in serving bowls and garnish with parsley

Per serving:

- Cal 484
- Fat 29g
- Net Carbs 3g
- Protein 22g

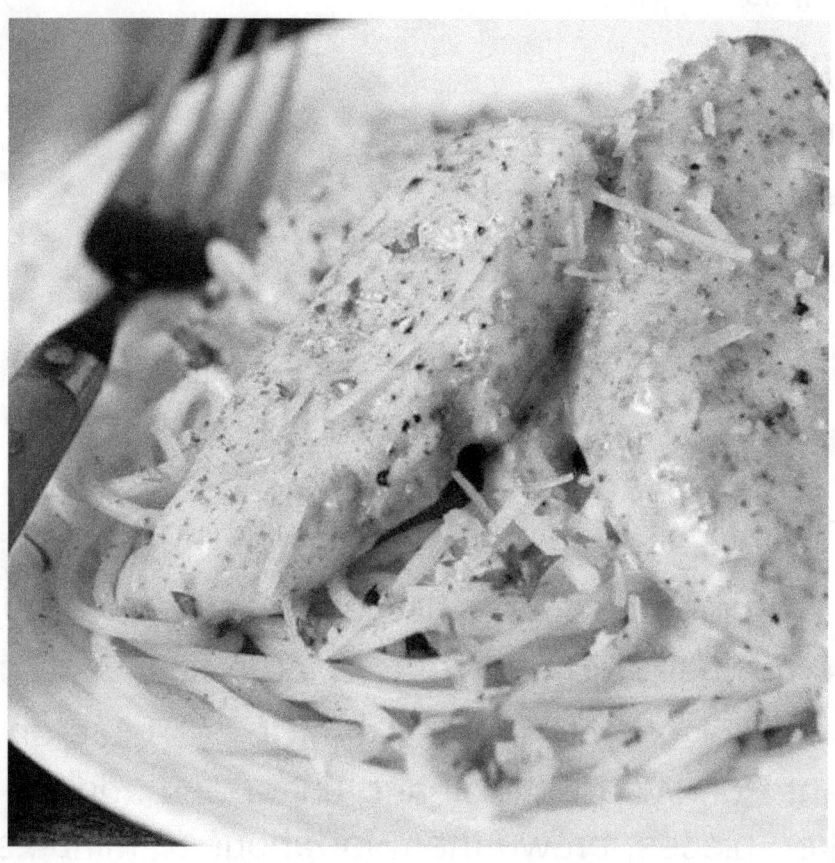

48. INSTANT POT NO BEAN CHICKEN CHILI

Ingredients

For 4 servings

- 1 lb chicken breasts
- 6 oz cream cheese
- ¼ tsp cumin
- Salt to taste
- white pepper to taste
- 1 cup chicken broth
- ½ tsp Cayenne powder
- ½ cup diced tomatoes
- 2 tbsp grated American cheese
- ¼ cup sour cream

Directions

Total Time: approx. 40 minutes

1. Place the chicken in the Instant Pot. Add the remaining ingredients except for the American cheese and sour cream.
2. Close the lid, secure the pressure valve, and select Manual on High Pressure for 15 minutes.
3. Once ready, do a natural pressure release for 10 minutes, then quickly release pressure and open the lid.

4   Shred the chicken using 2 forks. Stir and dish into serving bowls. Top with sour cream and American cheese.

Per serving:

- Cal 207
- Fat 12g
- Net Carbs 1g
- Protein 20g

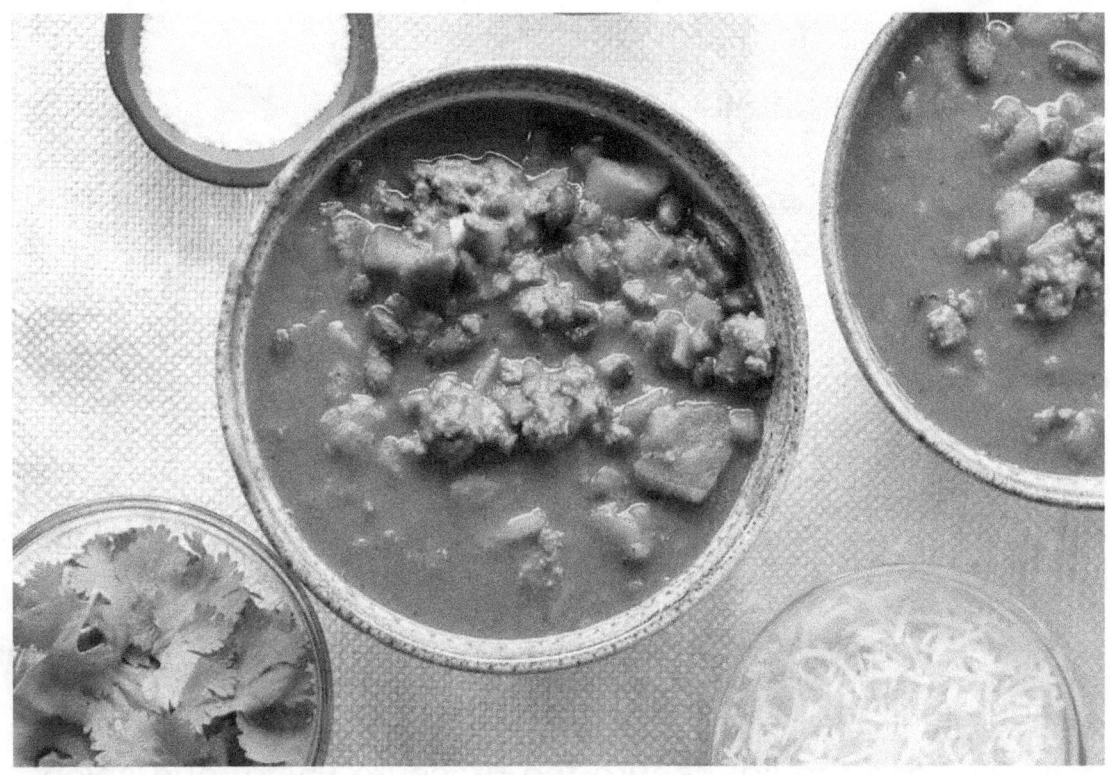

49. INSTANT POT CHICKEN SOUP

Ingredients

For 4 servings

- 2 tbsp olive oil
- 1 large carrot, chopped
- 1 large celery stalk, chopped
- 1 large white onion, chopped
- 6 cloves garlic, minced
- 1 green chili pepper, sliced
- Salt and black pepper to taste
- 1-inch ginger, grated 4 cups chicken broth
- ½ lb chicken breasts

Directions

Total Time: approx. 40 minutes

1. Turn on your Instant Pot and select Saute.

2. Heat the olive oil and add all the listed vegetables. Stir and cook for 3 minutes. Pour in the broth and chicken; stir. Close the lid, secure the pressure valve, and select Manual for 15 minutes on High.

3. Once ready, naturally release pressure for 10 minutes, then quickly release pressure and open the lid. Remove the chicken, shred it and return it to the pot.

4. Serve hot.

Per serving:

- Cal 146
- Fat 4g
- Net Carbs 4g
- Protein 14g

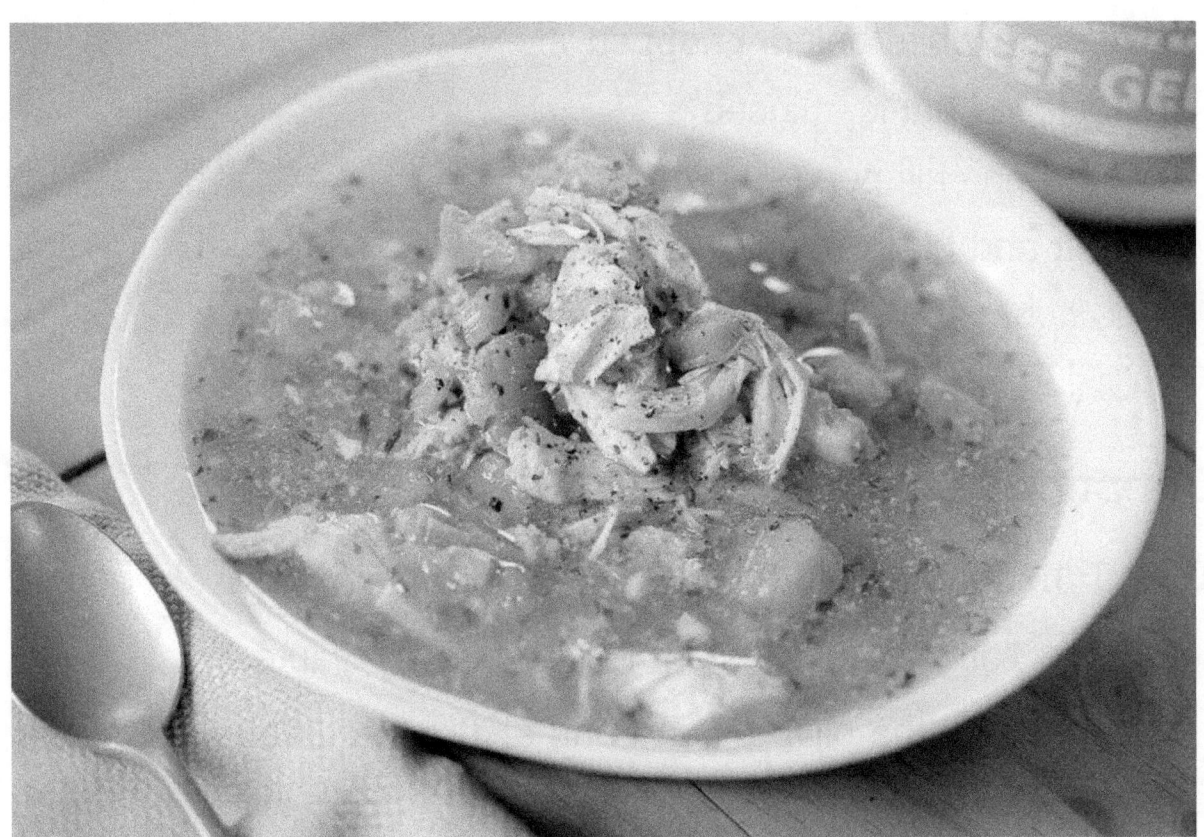

50. SOUS VIDE BUFFALO CHICKEN WINGS

Ingredients

For 6 servings

- 3 lb chicken wings
- Salt to taste
- 2 tsp garlic powder
- 2 tbsp smoked paprika
- ½ cup hot sauce
- 5 tbsp butter
- 2 ½ cups almond flour
- ½ cup olive oil for frying

Directions

Total Time: approx. 1 hour 20 minutes

1   Make a water bath, place a Sous Vide cooker in it, and set it at 144 F. Combine the wings, garlic, salt, sugar, and smoked paprika. Coat the chicken evenly. Place the chicken in a sizable vacuum-sealable bag, release air by the water displacement method and seal the bag.

2   Submerge the bag in the water. Set the timer to cook for 1 hour. Once the timer has stopped, remove and unseal the bag. Pour about the flour into a large bowl, add the chicken and toss to coat the chicken evenly.

3   Heat oil in a pan over medium heat, fry the chicken in the oil until golden brown. Remove and place aside. In

another pan, melt the butter and add the hot sauce. Coat the wings with butter and hot sauce. Serve.

Per serving:

- Cal 952
- Fat 65g
- Net Carbs 0.7g
- Protein 76g

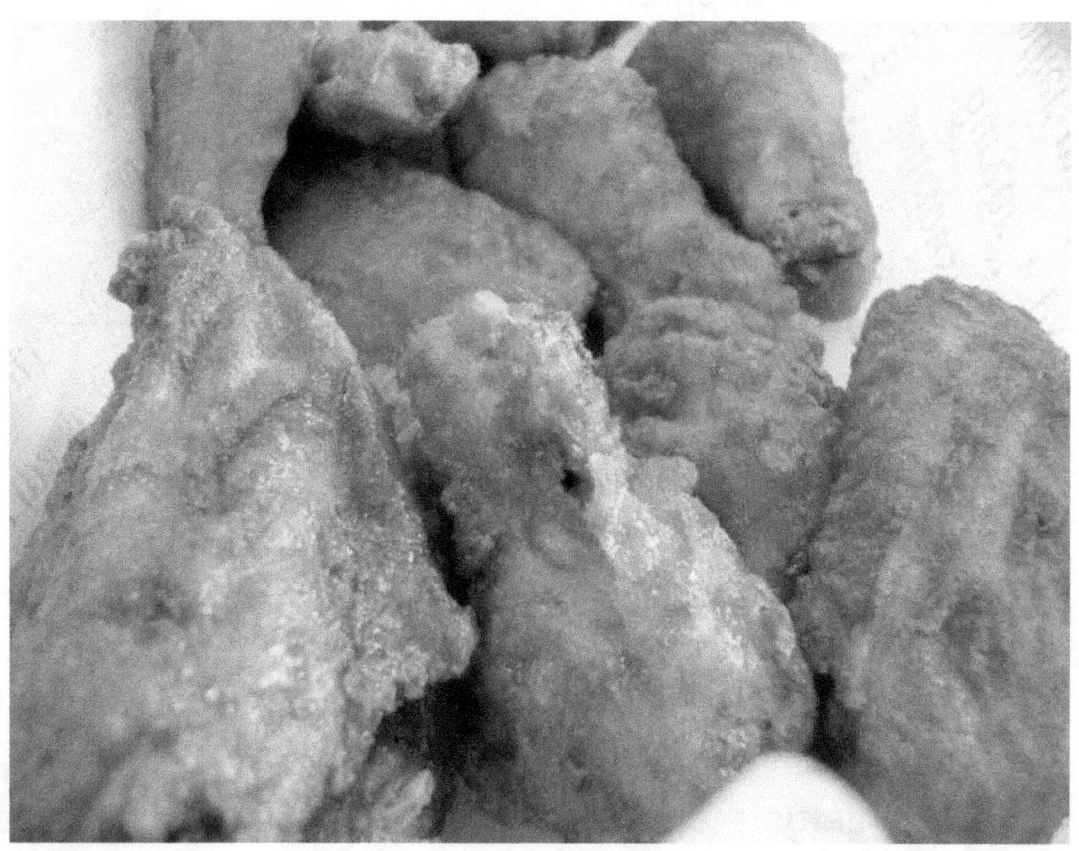

MEASUREMENTS & CONVERSIONS

	US STANDARD	US STANDARD (OUNCES)	METRIC (APPROXIMATE)
VOLUME EQUIVALENTS (LIQUID)	2 tablespoons	1 fl. oz.	30 mL
	¼ cup	2 fl. oz.	60 mL
	½ cup	4 fl. oz.	120 mL
	1 cup	8 fl. oz.	240 mL
	1 ½ cups	12 fl. oz.	355 mL
	2 cups or 1 pint	16 fl. oz.	475 mL
VOLUME EQUIVALENTS (DRY)	¼ teaspoon		1 mL
	½ teaspoon		2 mL
	1 teaspoon		5 mL
	1 tablespoon		15 mL
	¼ cup		59 mL
	⅓ cup		79 mL
	½ cup		118 mL
	⅔ cup		156 mL
	¾ cup		177 mL
	1 cup		235 mL
	2 cups or 1 pint		475 mL
	3 cups		700 mL
	4 cups or 1 quart		1 L
WEIGHT EQUIVALENTS	½ ounce		15 g
	1 ounce		30 g
	2 ounces		60 g
	4 ounces-		115 g
	8 ounces		225 g
	12 ounces		340 g
	16 ounces or 1 pound		455 g
	FAHRENHEIT (F)	CELSIUS (C) (APPROXIMATE)	
OVEN TEMPERATURES	250°F	120°F	
	300°F	150°F	
	325°F	180°F	
	375°F	190°F	
	400°F	200°F	
	425°F	220°F	
	450°F	230°F	

www.ingramcontent.com/pod-product-compliance
Lightning Source LLC
Chambersburg PA
CBHW081415080526
44589CB00016B/2539